Hello Beautiful,

Get Well Soon

When Hope and Healing

Are On The Other Side

G. Gigi Gilliard

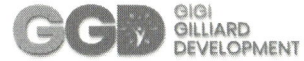

1st Edition

Library of Congress Cataloging-in-Publication Data is available upon request

ISBN: 978-1-7362657-2-7

E-book: ISBN 978-1-7362657-3-4

PRINTED IN THE

UNITED STATES OF AMERICA

Book Design

G. Gigi Gilliard & Larenz Brown

Senior Editor

Larenz Brown

Book Cover design

Olivia Pro Design

Book Front and Back Cover Photography

Orlando Smith Baugh / O.S. Baugh Media

Book Cover Hair and Make-Up Artistry
Ashley Wesley and Elleyse Wesley
3verlasting Impression

A special acknowledgment to:
My brother Andre Green and sister Milagros Lemus
Few have believed in my writing like you two!
I love you both. Thank you so much.

Team#GGD
Orlando, Sonja, Jules, Chi, Myra, Ommar,
Ayeshah, Melanie, Larenz and Lee
What ya'll need…courage, a heart, #steak? #BlackDorothy
Thank you **ALL** for *EVERYTHING.*
It does not work without ya'll.

Beverlyn, Stephanie & Lana
Steadfast and Unmovable- #Quad3 #RUReady!

Team#369MGM: Monica-Gigi-Myra
#BeyondTheDove #Hi…ThisIs6

Gamma Kappa Chapter Spring 1987
Bridget, Lauren, Ellen & Wendy
#GKLove #WeSTILLTogether #Ya'llKnowI'mPetty

Dr. Emily, Coach Amy Pittman, Coach Tamie Joyce, and Coach Michelle Griffith Davis
I am INFINITELY grateful! Thank you for the open windows!

Michelle Griffith Davis
Your love and friendship has guided my life.
You are a gift. I love you and I am so GRATEFUL!

Jeanine Erika Johnson-Smith
#SoulMating | #BFF2EHGKBUT | Enough said.

My sisters and my niece:
Altheresa Louise, Gida Mae, and LeAndra
When the niece is like the sister, and the Auntie is like the
mother, and the mother is like the sister, and *we all mixed up*!
#LOL **#Frankie'sGirls** #Chicken #FirstBesties #OnliestOnes

My Godfather and precious Uncle Bobby
You're my #1Buddy! I love you FOREVER.
Why do you have SO many nieces?? LOL

My Goddaughter Alahya
#RiseLikeACake, Goddie LOVES you…SO much!
And we are SO ridiculous! LOL

My STOLEN Goddaughter Brittany
#YouMineToo, I love you and Justin immensely.

To my Aunties, Uncles and FIRST COUSINS
Too many of ya'll on Mama *and* Daddy's side, but know
that I pray of all of you – DAILY. I love you so much.

Cousin Vanessa and James Wesley
Nessie, for loving me through every heartache and sharing
your children. THANK YOU. So grateful to you and Wes!

**The Gilliards, Middletons, Greenes, Plummers, Watleys,
Glovers, Johnsons, McKelveys, McHoneys, McNeils,
Linens, Poughs, Wrights**
I am nothing without my family. I love you all.

Pastor Kerrick Thomas and my Journey Church Family
I will never be able to express my full gratitude.
May God continue to bless you all.

My Parents
Frankie Gilliard & Sinobia Middleton-Gilliard
And of course, my Mama…

Sinobia "Shug" Middleton-Gilliard
I got it? YOU got it.

Love is the most excellent way.

****

*"A bruised reed he will not break,
and a smoldering wick he will not snuff out."*

- Isaiah 42:3

INSIDE

PREFACE

Have I ever told y'all the story about the 'dash'? I think a few of you may have attended one of my talks where I tell this story. If you've heard this before, please forgive me – but I think this will help you see my logic in creating this work.

First off, "The Dash" is not my story, so let me tell it to you the way that I heard it.

A Christian women's ministry leader, as part of her message to single Christian women during a Wednesday midweek service back in 2002-2003 - - asked us about what she called the 'dash.'

She went on to start her message by asking if any of us had ever visited a cemetery and taken a good long look at headstones. She asked, almost hypothetically, had we ever really studied the details that appeared on a person's headstone. After allowing the uncomfortable silence to hang in the air for a couple of minutes... she then went on.

She explained that one day while attending a funeral for a dear relative, she stood over the headstone of someone's grandfather (unrelated to her) and stared at the man's grave marker for some time. She went on to say that she noticed the following: that the man's name, his military service, his status as a husband, father, son, and soldier were all etched into the granite stone. She shared how she was mesmerized by the beauty of the marble of the headstone, and that although she was in the cemetery for the burial of a loved one, (reeling from her own pain brought on by the quiet sobs of her family), she became fixated on this one headstone. She told us that what captivated her most was *the dash* written in between the man's birth and death year.

She said that more than the man's birth year, or the year of the man's death, she was keenly drawn in that moment to the small dash that lay silently between the years of his sunrise and his sunset. She shared that it was in that moment she realized that the most important element on this man's headstone was this small symbol that represented all his years on earth. The dash, used this way, symbolized the life that was this man from the time that he was born, until the time that he died.

The dash made her wonder.

What had he done with his life? What had he done with those years represented by the dash? What had his life stood for? What had even her dear relative's life stood for? What was _her own life_ standing for? What would be her legacy? What would she leave behind? How would her life have served others? How would her existence have made a mark on other people in a way that brought _healing_ or _wholeness_ or _transformation_? For her, in that moment, on that cold Saturday morning as she stood over that marble headstone in that cemetery, the most important element on that headstone was the dash.

I love hearing a powerful sermon from an anointed woman of God. Now, there may be those of you who may challenge me with the _"but women should not preach"_ argument. Before we get uptight and all bent out of shape, please know that I am leaving that argument - - (for or against women preachers) - - to the Bible scholars. What I _do_ know is that the Bible teaches that women can _most certainly_ teach other women, and during this particular service, this woman-preacher was teaching, and imparting, GREAT knowledge.

It was during her message all those years ago, when she calmly and very quietly (in nearly a whisper) shared about the dash, that I knew I had to write you these things.

That very evening, I became fully aware that somehow, someway...*someday*, I was going to have to share about these very dreadful demons of emotional trouble and unwellness – particularly as it relates to grief and loss in my life.

I didn't have the language at the time.

I didn't know what was happening to me.

In fact, at that time, more than 15 years ago, I had yet to have the conversation that would change my life. It was a very specific chat with another spiritual leader that ultimately led me to realize how much help I needed – I share that story here. The night I heard about the 'dash,' I had yet to have that conversation that alerted me to how bad off I was.

Prior, I didn't know that I was depressed. I didn't know that I had general anxiety disorder. I did not know what grief syndrome was – – and quite frankly, I had never heard of these disorders.

However, I *did know* that I was off. Way off. First, I was crying all the time.

ALL.THE.TIME.

And look-it, for those of you who know me - that's saying something even for me because I am indeed a crier. I cry at movies; I cry at weddings; I cry over new babies; I cry when I say goodbye; I cry when I say hello ...I cry a lot.

I'm just set up that way. I've often, like many, believed it to be a sign of weakness, but during this period in my life, I found myself crying over everything – or nothing – *for nothing*. I would burst into tears for no apparent reason at all.

One morning, I was in the cafeteria of my job at the time. Early each morning I would order a small styrofoam cup of cream of wheat for breakfast. Enjoying the hot cereal in the cafeteria during the morning quiet, while the building was still empty, felt comforting somehow. On this one morning there was no cream of wheat available. As she always did, the lovely lady who worked the hot breakfast area cheerfully greeted me,

"Oh, hey good morning, Gigi... so sorry but we're out of cream of wheat today. If you look in the next tall silver warmer, you'll find some oatmeal though."

I stared at her as if she had intended to personally offend me.

The cafeteria lady stared back, unsure of what was happening. She asked if I wanted a larger bowl for some oatmeal. She seemed alarmed at my facial expressions.

I said nothing in return as tears pooled in the bottom of my eyelids. I could manage no audible or inexplicable response … but the streaming tears spoke for me.

"Oh no…oh no, honey…are you okay?"

Still not managing a reply, the tears continued to fall until I began to weep and weep loudly.

In the cafeteria – over cream of wheat.

I had begun to sob actually, uncontrollably so. It was stuff like that. These strange outbursts of emotion.

I was also edgy quite the bit. Jumpy, often very easily startled.

Born and raised in the Bronx New York, and certainly *very accustomed* to the occasional 'pop-pop-pop' sound of bullets (or sometime firecrackers made to sound like bullets), it made no sense that I was this jumpy all the time. If someone walked up behind me and I didn't sense them there, or they accidentally bumped into me without warning, I was jumping out of my skin.

I was also short. Meaning, I snapped at others easily over the smallest of things. There seemed to be brewing just under my surface this volcano of irritation, short-patience, and anger. The slightest spark would cause me to snap or bark or respond in a tone that was less than kind – and not my way.

Isolated, these behaviors may not seem a big deal.

Cumulatively though, it was odd conduct for me. Out of the ordinary and uncharacteristically suspect.

Then came the panic attacks. Small at first… times when I could feel my heart racing and my palms sweating. Then these "attacks" showed themselves much more prominently. My heart would feel as if it were beating out of my chest, my breath would become desperately short – almost like a wheeze, I would feel what seemed to be an irrational sense of being "trapped" and the feeling like "I can't find the door" would accompany all this. The crying, the jumpiness, the "snappiness," the panic.

All were happening too frequently, and 1 found that I had less and less control over these moments.

There were other signs that I'll share here as you read on. But for now, let's suffice it to say that these symptoms worsened in a short period of time. At the time though, I didn't have the presence of mind to understand them "as symptoms" and I ignored my bizarre comportment. As I saw that my behavior would draw unwanted attention, (for example, to my great embarrassment, co-workers, *whom I did not know*, gathered around me that morning in the cafeteria and tried to console me), I learned to mask my responses. I learned to clench my teeth in moments when someone asking me for a paperclip would fill me with murderous rage. I went to work, I built a business, I traveled, I became a successful corporate learning and development coach, I went to church, I had lunch with friends, showed great affection to my boyfriend at the time - - I learned to cope. I had almost faked myself out enough to believe that things "were better." But things were *not* better, and I was *not well*.

Four years after I heard the message of the dash, I was having lunch in a conference room with a co-worker. A very spiritual woman, who deeply loved God. This woman Cynthia became a mentor at work. Cynthia and I were becoming dear friends and I shared with her some troubling patterns I had begun to notice in my relationship. She was few years older and very wise - - and very direct. Up until this particular lunch, I had come to value her advice.

During our lunch she said,

"Gigi, if I am honest... I am very concerned about some of the things you've shared about your situation. I don't want to

overstep but I think that there are some things about this relationship that you should pay attention to."

I felt immediately uneasy because I wasn't ready to hear the truth. Cynthia went on.

"But more hon, I am concerned for your spiritual and emotional state. I've seen you react to some things – and some of the things you've shared make it obvious to me that you need some help. I don't think you are well."

What? Was she high? Was she buggin'? I didn't know her *THAT* well for this course of advice.

My defenses went *right* up.

"I'm fine." I shot back.

"You're not." She retorted. "You're not fine at all and I can see it all over you. Have you ever thought about seeing a therapist or talking to a professional? I think there are some things that God wants you to address."

Lunch. Over.

I was so offended that I quickly made an excuse to pack up my laptop and bag and return to my office. My friend tried to get me to open up again. As I packed up, she even apologized if she came across too strong. Yeah, I was good.

Smarting, (and lying), I told her I had forgotten I had to get to a meeting. She grabbed my elbow as I got to the door and made attempt again to apologize. I shot back a shady half-smile and told her I would call her later. I did not.

My office was on the other side of the building. I had to go down to the lobby and walk over to a far set of elevator banks to go back up to my floor. On the ride down to the lobby I was seething with anger. *"How dare she! She doesn't know me like that... and really, I shouldn't have been telling her my business! I don't know her either!"*

All excuses, because I knew she was right.

The next day when I got to my office there was gift on the small circle table in the corner across from my desk area. It was in a lovely yellow bag with bright yellow tissue paper. In it was a cup with a little girl on the front with these wild braids and the cup read, *"Get Well Soon."* There was a small note inserted from my friend Cynthia that read: *"I'm sorry if I hurt your feelings, but I'm not sorry about what I said Gigi...I do definitely think that you need to get well."*

I'm not sure why, but over the next few years as I cleaned out old boxes and would run into that cup from time to time,

(I held on to it), I couldn't throw it out. I would hold the cup in my hand and stare at the funny image of the girl with the wild braids (I was wearing braids at the time that the cup was gifted to me, so I did associate the girl with me).

A few years ago, I was moving into a townhouse I had coveted for a long time. This new home was a rare water-front property and signified an amazing shift in my life. As I unpacked my things, I found the *"Get Well Soon"* cup again and placed it where it could be prominently seen in my kitchen. As a housewarming gift, another friend, Minnette, had gifted me another cup that had on the front of it *"Hello Beautiful."*

Without thinking I placed the *"**Hello Beautiful**"* aside the *"**Get Well Soon**"* cup on the same shelf. I thought of neither one again, except for nice kitchen décor.

Nearly two years after being in my home, a set of troubling and unwanted circumstances had brought my world to a crashing halt. That same relationship, cautioned 12 years earlier by my friend, had ended in a dramatic set of events and emotions. The morning after our break-up, still reeling, I was standing in my kitchen, leaned up against my counter and crying out to God for relief from the pain I felt.

As I lifted my head from my prayer and blinked away my tears, I looked up at the shelf. The brightest ray of sun of shined gloriously and brightly on the shelf – but in a way that sent me a direct message. In that moment I saw the two cups together as a one message:

"Hello Beautiful, Get Well Soon."

That morning it was just me and God and the sunshine – and the work ahead. He had been trying to get my attention. He was trying to tell me that He although He did indeed find me beautiful, the admonishment was to **get well.**

To feel better, to get help… **to heal.**

In order to begin this process of taking care of myself, I found that I had to go back and uncover some things. Some pretty hurtful things. In the discovery, it just made sense to me to use my 'dash' to share what I had learned thus far on my healing journey with **_you_**…

Just in case it might help you with your own …

"get well soon."

HELLO

Chapter 1

What Princess?

E avesdropping is a skill.

No. That's not right. Eavesdropping is an **art**; and *a fine art at that*. Great eavesdropping in fact takes balance, concentration, dexterity - - and a discipline to control your breathing (so that you go undetected). I came to find that all of this is best perfected when you're 11-years-old and eavesdropping outside your parents' bedroom.

The delicate skill of extreme balance when eavesdropping proved necessary, because it just so happened that the floorboards under the carpet in front of our basement door were old and creaky. The basement door was just outside Mom and Dad's bedroom. If I was going to get close enough to hear every word he was saying, then I was going to have to stand still. Very still. I was also going to need, with precision, to be able to shift my weight from my right leg to my left in such a way to keep my body balanced.

I had to manage my stance 'just so'- - to prevent the floorboards from squeaking and giving me away. One wrong move with too much weight on one foot or the other, and I'd be busted for sure.

The way that my parents' home is constructed, the entry level has it so that you walk into the front door, walk past the living room and if you keep straight ahead, you'll hit the entry to the kitchen. Just there – at the apex of the living room and kitchen (off to your right), is a short hallway. At the end of that hallway was my sister Gida's bedroom. In the middle of the hallway to the left, was the full bath, and to the very right across the hall from the bathroom, was the door to the basement. Just on the other side of the door to the basement was a small alcove nestled right outside of Frankie and Sinobia's, my Dad and Mom's, bedroom.

In that alcove on one side, was a coat/linen closet. Across from that coat closet was a wall mounted with a full-length mirror. Now, if you were in my sister's room with the door open, you could look out into the hallway and then look into that mirror and see the reflection of my parents' bedroom. But standing in the hallway focused on balancing my weight, around the corner from the alcove, I had no vantage point. I couldn't see into his room, and I didn't dare peek around the wall into the alcove because surely, *I'd be caught.*

I had a rather small frame at 11-years-old, so the small space in the hallway in front of the basement door, just outside of the alcove was a sweet spot. If I didn't turn on the light in the hallway, (so that there were no shadows), my eavesdropping perch was perfected.

And I learned how to be perched in that spot each Wednesday.

Each and *every* Wednesday.

Not long after my 11th birthday, I noticed that every Wednesday evening between the time that we got out of school and the time that Mom came home from work, my Dad received a phone call.

He never let Gida, or I, pick up the phone on those days. (For those of you I haven't met yet, or for those who don't remember, Gida is my younger sister who grew up with me in the same house).

On these Wednesdays, he never rushed to the phone. It would take me some to time to realize that he *didn't* rush, because he would be sure to be sitting by the side of his bed because he would be <u>*waiting for this call.*</u> This revelation wouldn't come to me until much later when I realized exactly what was happening. However, I did notice the pattern. It was clear that a call came in every Wednesday evening right around the same time. It wasn't hard to figure that out. In part because he answered the phone barely on the first ring, and there was a tone in his voice that I didn't recognize.

On the one hand, his tone sounded might fatherly. Conversely, his voice also had a strange tilt. There was a certain 'singsong' in his phrasing that had just enough syrup to attract a very curious 11-year-old - - almost as naturally as a bee to honey. What's going on here?

Inquisitive and NOT to be lied to, I noticed the regularity of it all.

EVERY Wednesday? Same *time,* EACH week?

C'mon Bro.

Something was up.

I mean, I was a curious kid. Really curious. I was also pretty perceptive and felt things rather deeply. I realized early on that grown folk kept secrets - - and I knew enough to know that *"out-of-the-ordinary-behavior"* for adults could potentially mean that a secret was afoot. And my father's mysterious Wednesday calls made me *verrrrrrrry* curious about what the secrets he had going on - for sure.

Due to my level of "inquisitiveness," (and some of you would coin this just noisiness, but if you're going to start judging me only a few pages in - then we're doomed – so stick with me), my Dad, Frankie, had the chips stacked against him if he was looking to keep *whatever* this phone call was secret or private. He was out of luck if he thought he was going to get something past me.

There wasn't much I missed.

And seriously Dad? If you were going to be sneaky, I was going to need you to keep your voice at its regular octave, my man.

The inflection in his voice during these strange Wednesday calls became a dead giveaway. He sounded as light and as airy as a merry-go-round. His tone reminded me of a free-spirited kid with cotton candy and toffee butter popcorn in one hand, soda pop in the other, on a happy-go-lucky Saturday afternoon - - in an amusement park. It was sickening.

It was also quite obvious that the other person on the other side of the phone call was very, very important. Extremely. Important.

Whoever the "Wednesday-Phone-Call-Person" was meant a great deal to Frankie. A GREAT deal. This was no ordinary chit chat and judging from the loops in his voice this was no ordinary human. This was someone who made my Dad feel quite happy *on the inside.*

Oh yeah, … I was going to get to the bottom of this.

Furthermore, there was an ever so slight parental thing going on in his voice.

What was that about?

Every few sentences he would flip from *'happy-go-lucky-kid-in-the-amusement-park'* to very wise sage *'I've-seen-the-world Black man'* with a ton of gravitas in his voice.

I recognized the parental tone from the many times I'd heard him tell me to either clean up my room, wash the dishes, brush my teeth, or go to bed.

Yuppppppp… this was strange. Very, very strange.

He clearly wasn't talking to my Aunt Letha, or my Aunt Gracie, or my Aunt Toto (all his sisters). He wasn't talking to my Aunt Sandra or my Aunt Mena, (my mother's sisters). He wasn't talking to any of his sisters-in-law or any of HIS aunties or cousins (although I DID, at one point, think that he might've been talking to one of his two favorite female cousins:

cousin Susie or her older sister our cousin Janie). When I was much younger, I lived for a time with Susie, Janie and their three brothers as their Mom was my main caregiver as my young parents worked. Janie and Susie were like older sisters to me, but my Dad treated them both like sisters as well. Maybe these Wednesday calls were with one of them? Nah… I would know it. He wasn't talking with either of them. As a matter of fact, this call wasn't with any of those female relatives. I would have known (and, also, I'd eavesdropped on my parents' so much, that when he *was* speaking with any those women in our family, I knew the names, places, and topics to listen for).

Nope. No, no.

This was different. Way different.

This person was special, someone out of the ordinary. But gauging from the 'sing-song-y' thing Dad had going on, I deduced that the caller MUST be female. #Hmpf.

I was perplexed – but believe you me, I was dogmatic and determined in my pursuit to get to the ENTIRE bottom of all this.

So, Wednesday after Wednesday for nearly three months, I let Frankie go ahead and pick up the phone and didn't even try to bother to answer. We never had to worry about Gida running to get the phone because, as usual, my baby sister lived in a constant state of:

"I am unconcerned with you and involved in my own 7-year-old-affairs, thank you very much."

If you know her, you know what I mean. She cares about things, *kind of*. But only sometimes, and only a little, IF and WHEN she feels like it. She has always been the quintessential queen of unbothered.

When Wednesdays rolled around, and when his precious phone call came in, I <u>gave</u> him time to settle into his spot on his side of the bed (where the phone was on his nightstand) and waited until he got cozy.

Typically, he liked to have a late day cup of coffee and a cigarette during the call. Well, be relaxed why don't you.

The sun would be streaming through his bedroom window in that soft melancholy warm late afternoon way, and I remembered feeling the energy that this time was sacred for him.

Except that "I" then, was going to be a part of it too.

You got that right, jack.

It's interesting that I use the word 'sacred' because I don't know that at 11, I knew what that word meant. I actually don't think that the word sacred was even a part of my vocabulary or my lexicon at the time, but instinctively I knew that during this time on Wednesdays something spiritual was happening for my Dad. Almost like church. His behavior made me all parts curious and uneasy at the same time.

I was 11 and awkward and inquisitive; and not particularly fond of feeling uneasy.

So, when HE showed up for the phone call on Wednesdays at about 5:30 PM - - I was RIGHT there. Uncomfortably perched in my eavesdropping spot - every week. You and me Bud.

Resolute and committed to finding out WHO on EARTH my father was talking to.

And then one Wednesday it happened.

I heard it as clear as a bell.

Even as I share these words with you, I can hear it in my head, and I thought to myself *"Hmmm. Oh. Now we REALLY have a problem."*

It went a little something like this:

"Well Princess, did you do the best you could? Do you believe you gave it your all and your best shot? Was there anything else you think you could have done differently?"

All said in the 'merry-go-round-cotton candy-butter-toffee-popcorn-we-so-happy-go-lucky-on-a-Saturday-afternoon-in-the-amusement-park' voice.

But honestly, in this moment, I cared nothing about his tone.

He used the fighting word: **Princess.**

Princess? *WHAT* Princess? WHERE was there a Princess? What is going on here?

Who the heck was he talking to?!?

I told myself to calm down so I could reason it out.

My younger sister Gida was in her room with the door shut. I've told you… Gida RULES the land of all of the world's unbothered souls. She would probably heave and straight vomit if he even *tried* to call her Princess to her face. She was 7-year-old at the time and she and Frankie had the typical seven-year-old and her Dad relationship - - they weren't necessarily "buds." Gida is stubborn and can be thick headed when she wants to be. In that, in so many ways she was just like him. #Just.

I believe early on in their friendship they both recognized themselves in each other and were like, *"yeah we're going to have problems since we both want to be the boss."*
As such, Frankie certainly wasn't referring to Gida as Princess and besides, she was in her room, with the door shut.

That would leave, you guessed it, *me.*

But oh no, CLEARLY, he wasn't talking to me because I was busy hiding in the dark hallway while he was on the phone using the merry-go-round voice. As a matter fact, I don't believe that up until that point he had *ever* referred to me as Princess - - and I know *for a fact* that throughout the latter course of my life he never called that term. Never. He had a whole other nick name for me. So, apparently, the "Princess" was *NOT* me.

I was undone.

So not only was this individual getting deep parental guidance about "trying your best" and affirmation questions like: "*did you do well*?," (and please, let's not forget the merry-go-round voice), but now there was the audacity of this Princess business.

Are you kidding me?

WHO in the name of all things 11-years-old could he have possibly been speaking to?!?!

Who was this Princess? Was it one of MY girl first-cousins? Our extended family is so large, with both he and my Mom having nine siblings a piece – it certainly could have been any one of those girl cousins. And also, he did have a coworker named Ed, and I think that he was Ed's daughter's godfather.

Was it her?

I didn't think so though because she was still an itty-bitty-thing, so Dad having weekly convos with his two-year goddaughter this way didn't make any sense. The suspense was driving me nuts and this befuddlement had to end.

Not long after the 'Princess' incident, I actually called up the boldness to ask him about it. I didn't have the constitution or the integrity at 11 to confess that I had been eavesdropping for three months, but I *did* have enough emotional maturity to understand that if I wanted to get to the bottom of this, I was *just* going to have to ask him.

The following Sunday after we had come from church, I mustered up said courage. I marched into the kitchen and asked him to have a seat as I announced that we needed to have a talk. I was determined to be a big girl and make him look me in the eye as I queried him. I planned out that I was going to ask about his day, then ask if he wanted any coffee and then I was going to go in for the kill.

"Daddy, can I talk to you about something that I have noticed?"

Immediately he smirked. I was known for dramatic antics, and he was not surprised.

"Talk to me about WHAT Gigi? What have you noticed?"

He was already all parts annoyed and simultaneously amused. This characterized our life together.

He knew me well and knew that I often made a big deal about nothing - *and everything.*

"Well Dad, I have kinda started to notice that on every Wednesday, I don't know -- maybe around five or five-thirty you get on the phone, and you talk for a long time with someone. It seems like you're very delighted when you speak with this person."

Saying 'delighted.' At 11.

Now, I had every intention of going further with my inquisition, but the look of sheer horror and panic on his face spurred me on. I thought to myself,

"Oh, so I 'am' on to something."

So, I DEFINITELY kept going:

"Dad who is that person you speak to on the phone on Wednesdays? Is that someone that we know? Is that your friend Ed's daughter?"

The chestnut brown color drained from my father's face as I pressed.

"So that somebody that you talk to on the phone - - that's a girl, right?"

He didn't answer but he looked away sheepishly.

Yes sir, yes ma'am. I was on to something.

"Gigi why are you standing outside my door eavesdropping in the first place? How is it that you know when I'm on the phone and when I'm talking to the person?"

Don't deflect partna. Answer the question, Dude.

It wasn't my way to outwardly confront my parents. Doing so meant certain death. These disciplinarian southern folks did NOT get down like that. They were strict and they were serious, and they left no room for disrespectful little girls in their home. We were to be always polite, deeply respectful, never talking back... And *certainly*, never challenging. But this was too significant, and even as an 11-year-old I sensed that. Consequently, in that moment I took my life into my own hands and pretended not to hear the question about my eavesdropping, and I went on to daringly ask:

"Well, who is it then?"... Who is she, because clearly, it's a girl? It must be because I heard you say 'Princess.' WHO is the Princess? Who-do-you-talk-to-on-Wednesdays?"

At this point my father looked as if he was really going to fall into his coffee cup. He appeared startled, off-guard, and agitated. Quite honestly in that moment I should have planned to become an FBI investigator because I remember knowing, with certainty, *that somebody ain't tellin' me somethin'* (insert red cussin' emoji) ... and I DID.NOT.LIKE.IT. Not one bit.

Frankie adeptly skirted the question and never answered me.

He was evidently more skilled in the art of concealment than I was in the art of interrogation.

Expertly, he quickly changed the subject, got me interested in something else - -

and that was... well, that.

For now.

Chapter 2

16

Eleven year old girls can be easily distracted. Before long, the wiles of childhood had begun to set in, and I soon forgot about my father's Wednesday calls and the mysterious and elusive Princess. It was just at this time that I had become *deeply* enamored with a boy in my sixth-grade class. I told ya'll about him last time we got together.

I was distracted by grade school love, and all this let Frankie off the hook with a temporary reprieve.

Besides which, the school year was ending, and we were about to make our annual trip to South Carolina. Every summer, my Mom, (along with her siblings and their kids) packed my sister and I up and shipped us off to be with my grandparents in the South.

I know I've shared with some of you that it was our yearly custom to travel down south every summer and spend the summer with some of our first cousins all summer long. We would leave generally the day or two after school let out, and we wouldn't return until just before school began again in the Fall. This summer was no different. School was out that June of 1979 and we were on our way to South Carolina to spend the summer with our cousins and my mother's parents.

The drive from New York City to South Carolina is a gruel of a 14-hour ride. As such, it wasn't unusual that my parents would stay in South Carolina for several days before heading right back to New York. South Carolina is the home state for them both. In fact, my mother's town sits about 10 miles north of one of the larger towns (Moncks Corner) in that area, which is just a short ride outside of Charleston. My Dad's town sits less than ten miles away from where my Mom grew up, so this meant that both could visit with extended family before going back to New York City. This had become a big part of the custom of dropping Gigi and Gida off in South Carolina for the summer.

It was to be expected then, that my Dad would have us get dressed up to take us "back-in-the back-there" of St. Stephen, South Carolina. His relatives lived off the main road of St. Stephen (his town). To visit with his mother's sisters: Aunt Jesse Mae, or Aunt Susan or Aunt Mabel (when those of my grand Aunts were still living) was akin to a live history lesson on life in the deep South.

As such, it caused no alarm when on a certain Saturday during our visit that summer, that Frankie in the middle of the afternoon, told my sister Gida and I to come take a ride with him.

"Girls," he said, *"get in the station wagon. We're going to drive over to Moncks Corner to pick up a few things and go visiting."* Going visiting usually meant that we were going to see our Grand Aunts. My Dad's mother, my paternal Grandma Sarah had passed away by then, and Frankie loved parading us in front of her sisters – his Aunties. This was normal. But on this particular trip to Moncks Corner, Dad had it in his mind that Gida and I needed extra-special matching outfits. Okay, cool. No

prob. My parents very often dressed Gida and I in the same little girl 'get up' - - just in different colors. So that day when we got to Moncks Corner, Frankie took us into Piggly Wiggly and after walking around for a few minutes he landed on two versions of the cutest little, short set. It was a halter short set. Mine was pink with white flowers and Gida's, in the exact same style, was light green with white flowers. The top was a modest little girl halter top, and the bottom was a darling set of matching shorts. After the purchase of our coordinated outfits, we left the store and headed back for my grandparents' - my mother's parent's - house.

We got back to my grandmother and my grandfather's house and all our cousins were out in the yard playing. *"Where y'all been at?"* My cousin Jazz asked.

"We're going visitin' tomorrow in St. Stephen and my Dad wanted us to get something to wear." Regular stuff.

No one cared and we went back to the business of playing and enjoying our summer with our cousins.

Like normal, we tuckered ourselves out that evening and were hot and dirty and sweaty by bedtime.

As we came into my grandparent's house for the night, Frankie called us into the room him and said, "*okay girls make sure you take your baths tonight, get right in the bed and go right to sleep. We have an early morning tomorrow.*"

This also wasn't unusual in the least with all the heat and the sand from the dirt road that ran outside my grandparents' house – it made sense that we would get cleaned up before bed. When looking back though, I see that Frankie had a plan. He wanted to make sure that we were ready in the morning nice and early and that we didn't disturb my aunts, my grandfather, and my other cousins. Doing as we were told, my sister and I took our baths and got ready for bed that night.

****

For as much as I always said going to South Carolina during the summers was difficult for me (primarily because I hated the heat, the bugs and absolutely hated the sand), I don't know that there is anything more tranquil or more grounding than a South Carolina

24

morning. The rows of fields that you could see for miles, the treetops, the expansive clear blue sky, the smell of morning dew and the faint whiff of tobacco in the cool of the air in a place that was usually so stifling hot – felt almost celestial.

This was my parent's home… the place where they had grown up. And yet, it was so much a part of our own identity, that it was our home too. It felt safe and familiar and defining.

Like, this is who I am… this is where I am from.

Just as the sun comes up, (if you were standing on my grandparents' porch looking out across the dirt road onto the property across the other side of the road and beyond the big grass field that lay on the side of that property), if you looked straight ahead to the trees in the distance you would almost feel like there was no world beyond those trees. The only thing that gave it away was the sound of the Amtrak train in the distance and although the tracks were well hidden beyond those trees, you knew that the Amtrak train was coming from *someplace* on its way to another.

Nothing like those mornings.

Frankie did indeed get us up that morning, well before anyone else. It couldn't have been even 6AM yet, as the sun was just beginning to peak out. The roosters were crowing, and the cicadas were doing their morning clicking, but everything else was eerily quiet. Except for the occasional chicken strutting across my grandparents' front yard, there was no movement.

Dad came in our room and put his finger over his mouth as if to gesture that we should be quiet as we got up. He helped us out of bed and with his finger still over his mouth, he motioned that we should remain quiet as he ushered us into the bathroom to wash our faces and brush our teeth.

We noticed that on my grandmother's kitchen table were pre-made bowls of cereal and glasses of orange juice laid out for our breakfast. Now THIS was strange. We never did this in the summertime. We *never* ate without our cousins.

This morning felt different all of a sudden. This was very, very different. When I talk to Gida now about the memory of this day, she says she doesn't remember the cereal, or the quiet blissful South Carolina morning – but she *does* remember that we didn't eat breakfast with my cousins.

Something about *that* felt off.

It was as if we had our own special mission and that something strange was about to happen.

Quickly, Frankie got dressed, but he had taken his clothes out of the room where he and my mother were staying, and he made us get dressed off in another side room so that we didn't disturb anyone.

Even after we were dressed and began to make our way to the car, he kept his finger over his mouth, and he kept saying in a whisper *"okay girls let's hurry now we don't want to be late."*

Gida, seven-years-old and typically uninterested in adult antics, somehow had the presence of mind to ask, *"Aren't you going to wake Mommie up, is it Mommie coming with us?"* Frankie didn't look at her as he responded, he was lacing up and tying his sneaker. While looking down and doing so he said,

"No…no… your Mom is going to get her rest. This trip is just for me, you and Gigi."

Uhmmmm. Okay Dad.

He hurried us out of the door down the steps of my grandparents porch and into the backseat of our station wagon. I remember him turning the key in the ignition gingerly as if by turning the key slowly it would muffle the wrath of the engine somehow. Against the silence of the South Carolina morning, the car turning on sounded louder than a bulldozer. Nonetheless he slowly backed out of the front yard, and we headed north on the dirt road towards St. Stephen.

Before we even got a half mile up the road, Frankie looked in the rearview mirror to check on us sitting in the backseat. Gida had already begun doze off to sleep. Still really a little baby in some ways, her eyelids woefully lost out every time there was a nice car ride. And Frankie had gotten us up with the chickens. She was still so sleepy and in moments she was out like a light.

Oh… but not me. No Ma'am. No Sir.

What's happening here? Where were we going?

My 11-year-old Spidey senses were way too heightened to sleep. If we were just going to visit Aunt Mabel or Aunt Jessie Mae or Aunt Susan - - surely Mama would've come with us. If we were going to visit one of Dad's other relatives, we would have gone in the afternoon or in the evening time, as a whole family - - wouldn't we have? **_Where_** were we going? Why so early? And *WHY* were we going without Mama?

The answers were soon to follow.

Frankie had a good skill of keeping his eyes on the road ahead of him and having a conversation with me through the rear-view mirror. As Gida's car breathing swiftly turned into a child's soft snore, he said to me "*Hi,*"… as if that were the first time he was seeing me that morning.

Hi, yourself is what I wanted to say.

"Hi." I responded, eyebrows arched and then PROMPTLY followed with the question,

"Daddy? WHERE are we going? How come Mommie didn't come with us? What is going on?"

He told me many times later on in life that as he prepared for that moment, he always knew would have to deal with me.

Me especially.

My father's next words would change our lives forever.

"So..., so...you know the person you asked me about that I speak to on Wednesdays? You know when you're standing outside my bedroom door listening to my conversation?"

Wait! How did he know? He KNEW I was there?

I was ridiculous.

OF COURSE, HE KNEW I was standing there. In that brief second, I felt only fear and panic rise in my heart. I thought I had been so careful. How could he possibly know? I had been so proud of myself and my eavesdropping prowess! Also, he never let on that he knew I was standing out there. Do I lie? Frankie and I had just been through a whole thing about me lying about this little boy that I liked in my fifth-grade class. Cory Peterson was the cutest boy in our class and for whatever reason he had taken a liking to me. I was so smitten with Cory that I orchestrated this ruse to get he and I to sit next to each other in our fifth-grade math class. It just so happens that the Catholic school nuns didn't allow girls and boys to sit next to each other, which just meant that I would have to orchestrate sitting next to Cory in a caper. Cory then had the audacity to ask for my home phone number. He called the house one night when we were on our way out to my piano lesson and even though _I_ answered the phone and tried to play it off, Frankie figured out that the phone call was for me – from a little boy! This was highly problematic you see, because Frankie had a rule.

Shoot!

This Dude had so MANY rules, that it was hard to keep up...but his main rule was that no daughter of his was going to entertain a boy _on any level_ until we were 16.

We had to be at least 16 years old before we could even openly say out loud that we liked the boy - - let alone have a boyfriend. Furthermore, my Dad constantly threatened to move the age limit to 18. But to my knowledge, at last check... we had to be 16 to be involved with boy. No negotiation, no discussion, no nothing. 16 or no boys.

This became situationally challenging for me and Frankie, because as he and my mother quickly found out... I apparently came to this earth to do three things: (1) make friends, (2) give hugs and (3) find and fall in love with boys.   And I was serious about my missions.

I was a quirky, ill-fitting fifth grader, and Cory Peterson at that time, was the cutest thing going and there was no way on God's green earth that I was going to pass that up. I could care less that I wasn't yet 16. I gave Cory Peterson my phone number and he called, and I got busted. To make matters worse I concocted a very elaborate story about how and why Cory got our home phone number. Frankie investigated my tall tale, found all of my untruths, and PROMPTLY beat my tail.

Which he followed up with this whole long conversation about boys, about lying and about obeying his rules. It was a harrowing ordeal that exposed all my sin. This escapade happened the year before, certainly well before the time that I was supposed to have a boyfriend. We had just gotten past the whole mishegoss, and Frankie had forgiven me it seemed. He was my Bud again and I didn't want to get in trouble for lying anymore.

So, I answered honestly.

"Yes, I have been eavesdropping. For while. I have heard you on the phone with someone. That's why I asked you about it that day."

As he continued to drive us toward his hometown of St. Stephen, he also continued to manage to keep my gaze in the rear-view mirror. He smiled and smirked at me and said,

"No, you asked who the Princess was. And you asked me who I was on the phone with because your nosey behind stood outside my door listening on purpose."

Fair.

He was in a full grin now, so I knew I wasn't in trouble necessarily, so I responded confidently:

"Well… yeah. You did call the person a princess. Who were you talking to? Gida was in her room and I… I… you know… I was kinda…you know…standing nearby. "

"Standing nearby, huh…" He chuckled out loud.

"Yes, I was standing nearby, and I heard you on a lot of weeks, always kind of at the same time talking to this person and you seem really happy to talk to them. And then one day I heard you say Princess… you never told me who you were talking to?"

I treated Frankie like I was his boss, and he was late on deliverables.

As I searched his face in the rear-view mirror, I sensed that he was stumbling for words.

Finally, he just came out with it, and said

"Gi, I have something to tell you. Are you ready?"

As if on instinct Gida opened her eyes right at this point. I remember clearly as I share the words on this page that my younger sister wasn't paying more attention to the information that my father was about to deliver, then she was on my face and my reaction.

Over the years as we've talked about this incident, and in my mind's eye I can clearly see that she was less interested in what Frankie was saying and more curious about what was going on with me.

Personally, I was riveted. Ready for what, I thought?

"What do you have to tell me Daddy - - I can take anything."

Frankie was struggling.

Wow… This had to be big.

He went on, "Well… *well… what I wanted to tell you is that you have a big sister."*

Blink.

What?!?!

A big sister? What?!

Where? How? Where is she? What is he talking about?

At this point I had lived a decade, (and some), on this earth and it seemed inconceivable that there was another human being in the world that could be related to me as close as a sister and we did not live in the same house - - I remember thinking that. My mind was blown, and I wasn't comprehending exactly.

I had MANY questions.

I sat up closer in my seat, putting my chin on back of the front seat of the station wagon so that I could quiz him properly. "D*addy, what are you talking about? How could we have another sister? Nobody lives with us... but us.*"

While I promise you that I can remember this moment with crystallized precision, I don't exactly know how to describe the expression that was on Frankie's face. On one hand it was one of enjoyment as he watched me unpack this news. But it was also one of trepidation and fear,

... as he watched me unpack this news.

Poor Frankie.

"Yes, you see before me, and your Mommie got married I was with another lady."

Blink again.

How do the kids say right now on the Internet?

Dis tew much.

"Another lady? ... You mean, you had another wife? Do you have another wife now?"

My father burst out laughing...

"No silly, I don't have another wife. I don't have another lady this was before me, and your mom got married. It was about five years before we got married and you came along. But before you guys, I had another lady in my life and me and that lady had a baby."

My mind was young. It made NO sense.

"So... so...you have a baby?"

In later years as a definition of our friendship Frankie and I would talk about this moment in great detail. As a young adult he shared with me how much it tickled him that I was trying to piece this thing together. He confessed to me as well though, as we talked about it in later years how he regretted the decision to wait until my sister and I were older to tell us that we had an older sister. On the one hand he and my mother thought it was best to wait to tell us until we were old enough to process the information. But he also shared how much it pained him that morning that he was going to introduce us to her, because of how confused I was.

He wondered how this would affect my relationship with her going forward. He wondered how Gida would receive her. It was crucial to him that I, especially, got the understanding of what was happening.

He was counting on me to be the bridge between my little sister and my new older one. Well, she wasn't new - - she had always been there. But she was about to be new to us. He knew that Gida was too young to put it all together at seven years old, but he believed – he hoped - that I was going to bridge the gap, get to know my older sister and be able to explain all the details to Gida so that she would understand.

That meant *getting me* to understand this very grown-up concept - and why they had chosen to keep it from us would have a lasting impact on both my sisters. In seconds I went from being the older sister to Gida, to now the middle sister responsible for being a bridge. In those later years and in our later conversations he helped me to understand that being the middle child had a lot of responsibility to it and he was counting on me.

Great. Thanks. Didn't sign-up.

"Oh, I think I get it. You and the lady had a baby <u>a long time ago</u>."

He was staring at me in the rearview mirror marveling at how my 11-year-old mind was piecing this whole thing together like a modern-day soap opera… of which I was a character.

"Yes, that's very much what happened, Gi. As a matter of fact, it was 16 years ago that this happened. She came along before I married your mom and before you were born."

Wait… wait…wait…

Hold up. Hold the phone.

Hold the WHOLE the phone.

Wait one cotton-pickin'-minute.

Did he just say *16 years ago*?

Is he *actually* telling me that she 16 years old?

Oh, hang on. Let's get confirmation.

Did we hear this correctly?

"Daddy. What did you say? How old is she… exactly?"

I didn't ask her name… I didn't ask if she knew about us… all of that was peripheral and highly irrelevant.

I think he said she was 16.

"She's 16," he replied.

And in that moment my entire world was set right and in motion.

"So, you mean to tell me that I have an older sister who is 16? Is that what you're saying? You're saying that she's 16 years old?"

This could only mean one thing.

I'm really not sure how my father managed to keep his eyes on the road because I can hear his belly laugh on the inside of my soul as clear as I'm sharing this with you. Frankie let out such a gut level exhaled deep holler. He knew what this information meant, what's more, he knew with this information meant *to me*.

But there was more data to gather.

I needed to get <u>*the most*</u> important information straight.

"So, wait. Dad, Does. She. Have. A. Boyfriend?"

My longing 11-year-old eyes bored into the soul of my father in that rear-view mirror. As I looked at him in the rearview mirror, I willed him to respond with the only answer that would suffice. Yeah, yeah, yeah. Fine. Tell me more about that fact that we have an older sister. Cool, Wonderful. You had another lady; and the lady had a baby… this was all before Mom. Got it.

What I am REALLY interested in though, is everything about the love life of this new older sister of mine since she is 16.

She was 16, the magical age of love and romance in the Gilliard household. The only appropriate response was that this girl had a boyfriend. From the door if she wanted to gain her big sister Girl Scout badge from me, I was going to *need her* to have a boyfriend.

That was the only way that this strange twist was going to ever work for me.

Frankie was openly laughing now, and he replied,

"Well, honestly I don't know Gi, but you can ask her. This is where she lives. We're here now."

This response was weak and unacceptable to me.

Isn't this the individual who you've been on the phone with week after week on Wednesdays? Evidently this is the individual who you have crowned the Princess. Am I right? Ain't she your friend? Did you not share secrets? Did she not _tell_ you? Did you not _ask_? You know she's 16 – how could you *not ask*? How on earth do you not have the information about whether or not she has a boyfriend? How are you going to drop this news to me on our way to St. Stephen, TO GO MEET

HER, and you don't have the most important data point in the story?

I was crazed.

I honestly don't care what you were doing before you got married.

Personally, I'm 11 and that's your business… Who cares? What I need to know, is how come you don't know whether or not this little girl has a boyfriend… that's all that counts here. That's all.

Looking back on this entire thing and now recounting it for you, my friend, I see what God did.

In order to make this thing palatable for me, in order to help me to digest the fact that I had an older sister, God gave me the information with a spoonful, no, a bowlful, of sugar.

She was 16. *Well, how 'bout that.*

Which meant that she could *possibly* have a boyfriend.

Sweet Jesus, this was awesome!!

It's a funny thing about memories though.

If you talk to my younger sister Gida about this moment, she will give you a hilarious recap of how this moment went down. She does remember us going to get our little outfits the day before, she also remembers us getting up early that morning before our cousins and my aunt and mom. She remembers the ultra-quiet ride because no one was out but the chickens and the cicadas. but mostly in this memory my younger sister - - remembers *me*.

She'll tell you that she remembers my incredible excitement. She says that it was coming off of me like rays of light. This sense of joy, this sense of enthusiasm, the feel of promise about this new individual that we were about to take into our hearts. The problem was that because she was a seven-year-old without the sophistication of being a great eavesdropper, she didn't quite understand that through all of this excitement - - she was getting a big sister too.

As she watched her already existing big sister, (me), react with total glee and maniacal anticipation at the prospect of a 16-year-old being in our lives, her seven-year-old mind processed that this big sister was just for... wait for it... me.

In other words, my baby sister in that moment, on that ride to meet our 16-year-old sister for the first time, conceptualized in her mind that we were on our way to *meet Gigi's big sister -* and not hers.

She didn't get it.

And my exuberance didn't help things. In her seven-year-old mind she thought, oh of course Gigi's happy. She didn't have a big sister like me. I've always had a big sister and now Gigi is getting one too.

Nice. Good for them.

It would take us years, well into the future, to figure out that for many years Gida had no idea that our new 16-year-old big sister *was her big sister as well.*

She just thought what a nice day for Gigi, she's getting her big sister, I already have mine. So quite frankly I'm completely disinterested with this entire affair. And she also wasn't quite sure that leaving early in the morning and not telling my Mom where we were going would bear well... for any of us.

****

We had arrived now though, and it was time to meet our 16-year-old big sister.

Before long we were pulling into yard where my sister's grandfather lived. We were visiting her at her grandfather's house. I was so focused on the fact that she was 16, I had no time to be nervous. Oddly, though, as we pulled up to the door, (which strangely, I remembered for the first time as I was writing this to you), I do remember feeling a slight sense of jumpiness in my stomach. It was quickly overshadowed by the fact that the girl was 16 and I had information to gather. But I did have a stomach full of butterflies.

The energy in the air was... I will say electric, but also strange and exciting... like something brand new. It was as if we were about to step behind a curtain that all the adults in our life had been behind already. It was as if there was another room that made up the square footage of the house that was our lives. But this was a room that although it had always been there, we had never seen before and here we were, about to open this door.

As Frankie knocked, I remember that a very dark-skinned lady opened the door, and clearly, she knew my Dad.

"Hey Frankie, ya'll right on time. Y'all come on in. Oh, are these the other girls?"

Other girls. I didn't like that.

I remember this because the lady's eyes scanned my little sister and I up and down. She wasn't exactly welcoming, but she wasn't necessarily unfriendly – she actually didn't have much to say. She ushered us into the foyer, and I think we made a left down a small hallway. We were then ushered into a room that seemed to be a family room or den. In the corner, there was an older gentleman sitting in what appeared to be a recliner chair.

Dad went over and shook his hand and *"hailed him"* (which in the South is essentially the way we say he greeted him).

I remember that their exchange was extremely polite, but I also remember that it was a very chilly exchange as well. The older gentleman remained in his recliner and sat in that corner of the room while my sister and I sat across on this very beautiful brown couch.

The room was full of mahogany and deep brown colors, with blankets thrown over the back of the couches and chairs. On the far wall from the main sofa there was one full wall of shelves that held all kinds of books and Bibles and church hymnals and pictures of apparently all the people of this family. There were framed pictures of young black women in high school and a number of prom and graduation pictures along with some other family photos. There was a TV playing that was almost off to the side of this other gentleman.

Gida found a seat in the corner on the far side of the coach almost directly facing the older gentleman. He seemed to take a liking to her almost right away and asked her if she wanted to watch cartoons. She excitedly shook her head in the affirmative, and he turned the channel to whatever cartoon was playing. He and my sister both became engrossed in the cartoons together like two old friends.

Meanwhile, my father nervously sat down on the large brown sofa. The couch was a brown fabric that was really super soft, and it was positioned underneath a picture window across from the side of the room with the older gentleman sitting in his recliner. My dad sat in what seemed to be the middle of the sofa, I was sitting immediately to his left, and further left still our little sister Gida was sitting in a chair positioned just off of the side of the sofa; I was sitting between she and my dad.

As we sat, the room became uncomfortably silent. Like I mentioned it was obvious that my father and the older gentleman knew each other, but they exchanged very few words. It also became obvious that we were all waiting for someone.

To pierce the silence, the older gentleman said something,

"I don't know what that baby in there doin'… We told her ya'll was gon' be here round 'bout 7:30. That girl know she slow."

That girl.

That must be her. Who else could he be talking about?

That must mean that I was about to meet my sister.

Just then I noticed that Frankie was shifting in his seat. He started shuffling a little bit on the couch. He straightened his jean pants a little bit and he kept looking at the opposite side of the room towards the door. He was waiting for her too and he was nervous. Interesting.

I remember being fixated on his behavior. I was fascinated to see how important this was to him. I, too, was also filled with this indescribable, inexplicable, cacophony of feelings like wonder, confusion, excitement, and nerves.

I mean, let's not get it twisted. The girl was 16 and all... and there would, for sure, be the matter of finding out whether or not she had a boyfriend. Without question this was *first order of business*, you do understand that?

But certainly, something else was going on with me as well.

I didn't quite know what it was at the time, but I was about to find out. Because just then as I was becoming aware of my own emotions (too young to give them any language), I heard a sound that I'll never forget hearing in my life, and I don't know if I'll ever hear it again. It was something like the cross between a wind chime, the voice of a little songbird, ...and a giggle.

It was the sound of my older sister coming down the hallway. She was obviously laughing and talking with someone on her way into the room to see us.

Hearing the sound of her voice yet not seeing her, was striking because there was something astonishingly familiar about it. I know now that she sounded a lot like him, she sounded a *great deal* like him - - and that's what I recognized. I wasn't going to be able to process that right then, but I would come to figure this out much later on.

And then, ...

like the entrance of a Queen to her court, almost the way that a free-spirited little bird lands in its favorite tree... my older sister entered the room.

It would be way too dramatic to tell you that I thought that there was a halo around her head and angels singing, so I won't write that and be all MGM and Walt Disney about it...

But... There... Was... Something... Magical... About her.

She was lovely.

Beautiful and pretty and chocolate, and so lovely.

She had the height of a 16-year-old but generally she wasn't very tall. She had a smile that I had only seen in other place before my life...

And that was on my father's face.

Immediately looking at her face, and seeing this wide ear to ear, tooth filled happy grin, I knew. I knew with certainty; that this was Frankie's daughter. In the few seconds as she entered the room my brain was making the connection between the two of them. In that moment it was less about her being my sister and more about her being *his daughter*.

She bounced into the room with the energy of a typical teenager.

And then I heard it… "*Daddy!!!… Hi Daddy!*"

Waittttttt…wait…wait.

What's happening here?

Who is she talking to? This *guy*? This is *her* Dad? How?

Don't judge me. I just said I realized that she was his daughter, but I really didn't get it. I know he told us in the car that she was our sister. I know he prepped us to meet her, but I wasn't ready for this. If we had an older sister, HE had *another* daughter. And in that second, I put it all together. Well hello Wednesday call.

This was why the calls created that funny sound in his voice. That carefree sound which sounded half like a kid on a merry-go-round and half like a parent.

Oh, I see.

THIS is the Princess.

Well, hello Princess.

I guess.

Aside from her wide and blinding smile which was, without question, my father's number one physical characteristic - - she had the skin of a dark milk chocolate candy bar. She literally looked like a walking Hershey's bar. I had never seen a girl so pretty. Never. She had on a pair of cut off jean shorts and a T-shirt and she was effortlessly adorable. More than adorable she was really gorgeous - - like model gorgeous.

Before she went over to him though, she sort of stopped in the middle of her tracks as she entered the room. She looked over at the man in the corner and I think she said something like "hi granddaddy," and then she immediately turned her attention to me and Gida.

"Daddy... Is this them? Are these my sisters?"

I think at this point Gida maybe looked up from the cartoon, (maybe), and then our sister looked back and forth between the two of us. First to Gida, then back to me... then back to Gida and then to Dad. *"They are so cute Daddy!"*

There it was again... She called him Daddy.

Got it.

This was going to take some getting used to.

And then I wasn't ready for what happened next...

Out of nowhere, she jumped into Frankie's lap and threw her arms around his neck and said,

"Oh, Daddy I miss you so much!"

Oh. So, they've seen each other. Wow.

Sure. They'd been on the phone every Wednesday... but for how long? 16 years? Must be. Interesting!!

The action of my older sister jumping into my father's lap played out like some slow-motion scene in a movie. While I was immediately smitten with how pretty she was and her exuberant friendly personality, simultaneously, the computer that was my 11-year-old brain was trying to figure this all out.

I was feeling something.

A brand-new emotion.

An emotion I don't think I'd ever felt before.

I think the fledgling beginnings of this emotion were creeping in my heart as I was doing all that eavesdropping outside of Dad's room, (while he was on the phone clearly with the Princess – who has now been revealed), but the emotion wasn't full-blown until *jusssttttt* that moment.

I was jealous.

I was confused and happy and excited and full of wonder about this 16-year-old beauty (we had yet to get to the full inquisition about the boyfriend but trust me that was coming) … but if I'm honest, for the first time in my life at 11 years-old I felt the sting of jealousy.

They had a relationship that was *obvious*.

And what was more obvious was that this relationship had been going on and my younger sister and I not only knew nothing about it - - we knew nothing *of her*.

She and Frankie loved each other. Whoa.

This was a lot.

There was a lot happening in my young mind and heart - - and I had a million questions. But as my sister sat on my father's lap and my 11-year-old brain began to compute that my father shared his love with another young lady who he called Princess - I was also concurrently coming to instantly love her myself.

She was like a Hershey's Angel. No wonder he sounded like he was at an amusement park! Her voice was fun, her eyes danced when she talked, she was excited, she was talkative, she laughed really loud... she was *just like him!*

Whoa. Okay, this is happening.

I do remember her giving us hugs.

I was so happy to hug her. She was so friendly in fact, she felt like an immediate new best friend, who automatically liked you and wanted to hang out with you. I remember her putting her two hands on my cheeks and her saying that she thought I was cute.

She said that a few times actually.

Even as she sat on Dad's lap, she would turn and look over her shoulder and she would say to Dad, "*they are really soooooo cute!*"

It was about right this this point when I noticed him - - noticing me.

I don't know if I actually remember this happening or if it was because Frankie and I had talked about this so many times throughout the course of our lives that this comes to mind. But he told me in much later years that he could see on my face that I was trying to figure things out.

He shared with me in my own teenage years, and then later as a young woman in my early 20s, that in that moment that he took us to go meet our older sister he realized…

Oh man, I'm going to have to deal with Gigi on this.

And he was right - - he had a lot of explaining to do!

The rest of the morning was really nice. We didn't have breakfast with my sister's family, but I do remember the lady who greeted us at the door bringing us an orange drink that tasted a little like Tang.

We drank our juice while my oldest sister, Althreasa (we call her "Trease," and her friends call her "Al") sat easily with us and we got to know each other for the first time.

For now, I was going to have to put aside my confusion and my wonder about her relationship with Frankie because it was time to get down to business.

"*Can I ask you a question?*" I started gingerly.

She looked over at me for the first time with a sense of happiness that she could answer a question for me. This is so hilarious to think about because she still gets this way when I ask her questions. Her eyes light up, and there seems to be almost a great delight in her that she gets to impart her wisdom to me.

"Sure!" she said, "ask me anything… let's get to know each other."

Oh, she was super friendly; super, super friendly.

How lovely is she.

I went in… *"Sooooooo, you <u>are</u> 16, right?"*

Just then I saw Frankie begin to smirk again. He loved remembering this moment and we talked about it very often. My oldest sister said, *"yup! I turned 16 in March."*

Great. Let's get to work.

"So do you have a boyfriend?"

Let's cut to the chase, please.

My heart was in my chest as I awaited her answer. If she said no, we were going to have problems. How could you be the whole Frankie Gilliard romance age, where we could <u>have </u>a boyfriend and you didn't have one. This would have been a travesty that I'm not sure we could have come back from. I really needed her to say the right thing here.

But alas exactly what I hoped would happen, happened. And then some. This wiry, precious wide smile came across her face. The kind of smile that only comes across the face of a teenage girl in love. I recognized it immediately and she was in. In that instance I forgave her and Frankie their secret friendship or relationship or whatever they had … and their private Wednesday afternoon calls (yes, yes… I know this is very selfish of me… I get that! Stop judging this whole thing jacked me up).

I forgave them in that instance because not only did she have a boyfriend, but it appeared that she was quite smitten.

Oh yes baby, she was a keeper.

"*Yes!*" she answered in a song, *"I do have a boyfriend and he's really cute."*
She winked at me.

Come on in here Lord, we have LIFT OFF!

Instinctively, I scooted over on the couch, and I made a wide space between me and Frankie so she could sit down. I patted the couch as if to motion for her to sit on down next to me so we can get into it - and oh, man-that we did.

"Sit...sit... please. TELL-ME-EVERYTHING"

I promise I think I felt a pair of rolling eyes from Gida in the corner, but I was focused.

I wanted to know everything... how she met him, how tall was he, was he handsome, had they started holding hands yet?! Did she know his friends, did he know *her* friends, what was his name, did he write her love letters??

Spill it out girl!!

Here's where I remember too I that there were things that a sister shares with you that you can't share with your Dad. I wanted, so badly, to ask her had she kissed him, but I was smart enough to know that I couldn't ask that in front of Frankie.

Oh, don't worry biscuits, I was going to get this Hershey Princess by herself so I could ask her had she kissed him. We sat on the couch with Dad to the right of us, with her Grandfather sitting in the recliner chair across the room, with our little sister sitting on the other side of us on a chair watching cartoons. We sank into that couch in that sitting room and jumped into each other's lives. As we sat, the morning sun was streaming in the big picture window right above the couch. She turned her body in such a way that her head was leaned against the couch as she was staring at me... I was sitting on the couch the same way and we were becoming friends...immediately sharing secrets.

We were discovering what it meant to be Frankie's girls and forever etched in our hearts that moment we knew that we would never be apart again.

Maybe we stayed for another hour or so. Surely, I don't remember that exactly, but I know that we talked a lot. She did spend some time with Gida also, but we know now that Gida wasn't entirely sure what was happening. What we know now as adult women is that Gida was having her own processing.

She wasn't necessarily thinking about the fact that Frankie had another daughter... She didn't quite care about that.

But like I told you, we did find out later on that Gida's 7-year-old mind thought that she was witnessing me, Gigi, her big sister... GET a big sister. In later years we would come to know that her seven-year-old thinking believed that everybody *only got one* big sister. So, in her perspective, she had hers already.

She didn't put together that this big sister belonged to her also. It would take us well into our 30s before Gida admitted that to us. I found it hysterical.

"How could you not know she was your sister too?"

"Gidey" (what we call her) would always retort, *"well the way that you were carrying on with her as if she was the greatest thing come down from heaven in a boyfriend basket, what else was I supposed to think? This seemed like your new big sister... You seem like you were in love... And I thought, good for y'all: nice. Enjoy ya-selves."*

****

The story of our sister Trease coming into our lives is paramount.

Later that summer she came back to spend a week with us in New York. I soaked up every moment asking her about her favorite subjects and her friends and what she wanted to be when she grew up, and if she was going to college, and what her favorite color was, and so much more. It was like I was finding a piece of myself that I didn't know I was missing - and it was exhilarating and fun and sweet and so affirming.

I felt wholly and completely loved and accepted for no reason at all except because I existed. I found that Trease had the same experience. Getting to know these little girls who loved her JUST for her. We had the business of having to figure how we shared Dad – but that would come later when things would get complicated. For now, it was just pure love, pure acceptance, and the feeling of full belonging.

It was the first time also that I can remember having an episode of separating from someone who made me feel so wonderful and whole.

After that week in New York, I became extraordinarily attached to my older sister. She was kind... so very kind. She was interested in us in a loving and full way and believe you me she had a lot of questions for us and Frankie as well. That week together was a time of bonding, deep bonding, discovery, and pure friendship. I'm not entirely sure how to explain what happened next but it's important that I start with this because this is the first time, I remember having this kind of episode.

On the following Saturday after she had been with us the whole week, we took her to Penn Station so that she could get on Amtrak and go back to South Carolina. For whatever reason, in part because I know that I had already learned to hate goodbyes, I began to feel a feeling of dread and intense fear throughout my body. I just didn't want to say goodbye, but the feelings were extremely heightened. Was I afraid that I would never see her again? Was I afraid that I would never feel this kind of full unadulterated acceptance again? Was I afraid that this new experience of friendship and wonder and closeness would never come to greet me again?

Was I afraid that something would happen to her? Did she have friends who would love her like her sisters did?

I didn't have the words then, but I now know what happened in the car on the ride to Penn Station.

As we were about to say goodbye to my newly discovered, *"boyfriend-ed,"* sixteen-year-old-Hershey-Angel-Big-Sister, something was happening. (By the way, for my petty participants, I was NOT ready to call her Princess; the way my jealousy was set up).

I was about to have my first panic attack.

In recent therapy sessions I have heard it labeled as anxious attachment style. I get attached easily, quickly, fully - - and anxiously. The anxiety, in part, comes from loving the good feeling of being attached to someone who treats you so well (and accepts you so fully) and being afraid that you'll never experience that again. Add in for me by the time that I was 11, I had already had opportunity to say a lot of goodbyes and I hated them. That's not right. I don't hate goodbyes *past tense.*

I hate them *now*; so much.

I had also, by this point, been bullied mercilessly and my older sister's acceptance felt like an antidote to that poison.

We got to the station, and I remember Dad unloading her bags and Gida waving goodbye. The fear and sadness that gripped me was almost crippling. I wanted to be last to hug her because I wanted to hug her longest. She was so sweet; she sensed my anxiety – and she lovingly wiped my tears.

"Hey, hey why are you crying?" And I was crying something serious at this point. You would have thought that we spent every day of our lives prior to that time together. Finally, a super pretty, really cool girl accepted me. For me. And in fact, she was my ACTUAL sister. What if I never saw her again? What if something happened to her? What if she didn't like me the next time she saw me? Would she be safe on the train? Who was going to take care of her on the ride back? Why did she have to leave? I hated this moment so much. I did NOT want her to go.

And I remember it like it was this morning.

Even as I write this to you the tears stream down my face which is so silly because I've seen my sister hundreds of times since that day over the last 43 years.

She's on my phone REGULARLY.

In my life DAILY. But even, right now, as I recall that moment of having to say good-bye to her, I can feel the etchings of a panic attack beginning to well up.

She remembers this moment too.

We recently talked about it. She teases me a little bit about it...but only a little because even after all this time it makes sad.

I was only 11, already quite anxious about losing folks, and I was desperately terrified of that... *for sure.*

It was indeed a panic attack, and the first of many, many more to come.

Hello, panic attacks.

Apparently, you are my new sibling too.

Chapter 3

Mr. Young Man

G etting to know our older sister was great. Over the next few years, we wrote and called Trease often and before long it was hard to remember *not* being in each other's lives. It was a good thing too. I was on my way to high school and SURELY, I was going to need help with ALL the boys I would meet there. *wink* Are you judging again? I told ya'll I was focused as a kid.

Grade schoolboys were one thing. But high school boys? Well, that was new and significant romance business.

The next three years went by in a blur. I suddenly went from an awkward 11-year-old middle-school kid, to a slightly *more* awkward 14-year-old high school freshman.

Frankie and Sinobia weren't sold on public school education, so they sent us both to Catholic grammar school, at which I had several amazing friends. One friend in particular was my best friend, Joyce.

For those who spent time with me last time, you'll remember her.

Joyce and I had been best friends since well before the sixth grade. We began our friendship as "walk-to-school-together" buddies as her house was on the way to Holy Cross Elementary, where we were both students - - but we became true sisters as young girls in every way.

The day after we put my sister on the train back to South Carolina it was Joyce who calmed me down during hours of 11-year-old counseling phone calls.

As a dear childhood friend, it wasn't unusual then when we started talking about what high school we would go to. On the Catholic grammar school circuit in the Bronx in the late 70s, the process for picking a high school was a bit like choosing a college. There was an admission test for Bronx Catholic high schools at that time and contingent upon how well you did on that entrance exam, you got to choose which high school you wanted to go to.

There were a couple of options for me; two of which were all girl schools… which, if you haven't figured out by now, were **not** options. Additionally, it had come to my attention that my first true love, (who besotted me in the sixth grade when he delivered my first inelegant French kiss in the tunnel of love on a class trip), was going to a prestigious high school in the North Bronx. I want to tell you that I made my choice for high school because of my redeeming and noble academic goals, but not so. I'd love to even be able to tell you that I picked my high school because I wanted to be with my best friend Joyce. But that also would be untrue.

No, no…

I am embarrassed to say that I made my final choice about which high school I would attend based solely on the information that my six-grade crush (who I was still madly in love with by the way), was going to said prestigious high school. It did not hurt that Cardinal

Spellman High School was one of the best parochial schools in the Bronx. I am a proud alum now, but not so proud to say that the reason why I selected Cardinal Spellman in the first place was because I was on a love pursuit. Please don't tell my mother - - and to all my fellow Cardinal Spellman high school alums forgive me, I was a whole mess. And ain't much changed.

Alas, as childhood romance goes my grammar school ex-boyfriend now paid me no mind in those hallowed high school halls. Not even so much as a passing glance except when he occasionally saw me on one of the three buses, we rode from the North Bronx back to our neighborhood of Soundview.

Almost daily I rode the bus with Joyce. We would meet up at a certain point in between our two houses and begin the three-NYC-buses-trek to school. We didn't have any classes together so it was rare that we would see each other during the day, but certainly by day's end we would meet up again so that we could embark on our long trip home. All first year in high school this was our process, and it was good to have a friend who I grew up with by my side as we navigated the tricky, and sometimes treacherous social waters filled with mean-girl creatures of the deep that occupied high school life.

Without a doubt, like I am sure many of you, we witnessed the sure formation of distinct social groups. Joyce and I had never paid much mind to the fact that she was Puerto Rican, and I was Black. However, high school life certainly drew the lines. There was the pretty girl group, the athletic girls, the smart girls, the Black girls, Latine/Latina/Latinx girls, White girls, rich girls, bad girls, good girls… and then us. One way that our social groups were defined was by who rode the buses to and from school together. Many of the Black girls that were my friends in high school didn't live in our neighborhood. This meant that as I traveled to and from school with Joyce, I often rode the bus with *her* friends who at the time were considered a part of the Latine/Latina/Latinx girls. Cool.

In the group of friends that Joyce hung out with there was one Latina that Joyce was extremely friendly with:

Margarita Maldonado. Margarita was a sophomore, extremely popular, very friendly, and always seemed to be the life of the party. Margarita lived not far from us, and for the most part, took our same route home on the bus. Margarita was also super pretty and a very warmhearted girl. She was quite popular and well-liked. I didn't really fit in with Joyce's friends, (not necessarily because I wasn't Latina, but more because these were *her* friends and not really *my* group) - - but Margarita was still very welcoming to me.

Half-way through our freshman year, as Joyce and Margarita were becoming closer friends, riding the bus home every day with Joyce meant also riding home on the bus with Margarita and her whole crew. Margarita was certainly the nucleus of their bunch, and she was known to introduce new friends to their circle - - and she was also known to matchmake.

There was this one Black boy (who was quite tall), who hung out with them from time to time. He was clearly Margarita's friend, and it was also clear that they cared a great deal for one another. I later found out that

Margarita and the Black boy had grown up together in neighboring buildings before she moved to a new neighborhood - - so they had known each other as really young kids well before high school.

The boy was a bit shy it appeared, and it also appeared that Margarita had an affection for shy people. She was motherly to some extent and seemed to want everyone – even at 15 – to be happy and taken care of. It also became apparent as I spent time riding the bus with Joyce's friends, that the Black boy was somewhat of an outsider himself in this group. As such, I could see that Margarita wanted to make sure that her friend felt comfortable. She often saved a seat next to herself on the bus for him, and they whispered and giggled amongst themselves often.

Margarita filled him in on the inside Latin jokes and would sometimes even translate for him if they began speaking in Spanish. It never looked like anything romantic was happening between the two of them necessarily, but it *was* evident that Margarita cared for him.

She also cared a great deal for Joyce. To us she was an upper-class woman (Margarita and most of her crew were sophomores), and I think she took a special interest in Joyce as she saw herself as a big sister. By extension, which meant that Margarita went out of her way to be nice to me. She didn't know me well, but she knew that Joyce was my best friend and that gave me all the credit and access I needed, to this fun family of teenagers.

Around March of our freshman year on one of our bus excursions home, I distinctly remember Margarita sitting next to the tall Black boy as Joyce, and myself and others, sat across from them. She and the tall Black boy laughed easily and were obviously giggling about something personal, but every now and again she would look up and catch my eye as they talked. I would quickly look away because I didn't want it to seem like I was all in their business, but when I would look back again, it wasn't Margarita who was looking at me - - but it was the tall Black boy. This went on a couple of times during this one certain bus ride, and I remember thinking at some point that they may have been talking about me; maybe not in a rude or malicious way, but something seemed to be going on.

As Joyce and I got to our stop, where we would transfer to our last bus route that day, I noticed that the tall Black boy followed us off the bus and to our last bus stop as well. Margarita also got off with us.

"Oh," I thought to myself, *"he must live in Soundview too."* As we waited for the last bus the four of us were at the bus stop.

Joyce remarked, *"Rita,"* (her nick name) *"why'd you get off the bus? You don't live around here anymore."* Margarita responded, *"no, Nena I don't, but my grandmother still lives in our old building and I'm going to visit her."*

So, at the bus stop stood: Margarita, the tall Black boy, Joyce, and me. As we waited for the bus, I noticed that Margarita looked at Joyce, and then Joyce looked back at her in this weird and knowing "*cat that swallowed the canary kind of way.*" What was wrong with them, I wondered? Everyone was weird as teens, so I shrugged it off.

As the bus pulled up and we got our high school bus passes out, Margarita tried in a very nonchalant way to casually introduce me to the tall Black boy. Only it wasn't so nonchalant, and it certainly wasn't casual or smooth.

"Gigi, have you met my friend?" I had met him.

Oddly, we had officially met some time back in our high school cafeteria as I ate lunch with the Black kids one day. He was close friends with the boyfriend of a girl I knew from the African American club. Almost simultaneously we both said, *"Uhhmm...yeah, hi we know each other."*

He smiled coyly and looked away.

I told you that Margarita's introduction was neither nonchalant or smooth because she paused for an uncomfortably long time after attempting to introduce us, and then started giggling uncontrollably. Joyce was shaking her head, but she was also stifling her giggles. What's happening here I thought? What could possibly be so funny? The bus came, we got on, we got some seats and that was the end of it.

We rode home and we each got off at our respective stops. I lived the furthest, so I was on the bus the longest, and as usual got off last. We all saw each other in school the next day and it was as if nothing had happened, and no one said a word – that was that.

For some reason, it would be sometime, months even, before I saw the tall Black boy ride on the bus with us again. In fact, I saw him more in the school hallway and in the cafeteria after our awkward "introduction." He always spoke, but he was always seemed so bashful and would look away after saying hello. I thought his shy act was precious. I liked shy boys too.

Before long, the school year was ending as the weather got warmer. Friday, June 11th, 1982, was a very warm and very sunny spring day. It's a day hard to forget.

Joyce and I were at the end of our first year, and we were looking forward to a fun and long summer break. On this day she said, *"let's just leave early and ride the bus together without all those people – just us two like old times."*

I liked Joyce's friends just fine, but I was thrilled for the opportunity to have my childhood bestie all to myself.

We stopped and got a slice of pizza, (as Bronx girls often do on their way home from high school), we talked easily about our plans for the summer and what we were going to be doing with our families, and Joyce also talked incessantly about this boy Raphael she liked. We talked about our grades and about being so glad that the school year was over. Cardinal Spellman had a rigorous academic program and we both needed a break. It was the perfect fun-happy-lighthearted-springtime-ABC-afterschool-special kind of day.

As we got to Westchester Square, which was the point we needed to take our second bus, we walked to the stop and there was the tall Black boy. All alone.

Joyce exclaimed, *"Oh look Gigi, look who's waiting by himself!"*

I saw him.

As we got closer to stop, the tall Black boy waved at Joyce, and because of Margarita they had become good friends. *"Hey Joyce… wassup girl?"*

Long pause.

"Hey… Gigi."

Boy-incapable-Gigi strikes again… and all I could manage was a measly and inaudible *"Oh, hello."* Out of the corner of my eye I saw Joyce smirk and to this day I promise she giggled quietly. And like a cheerful cruise director orchestrating on-deck shuffle-board activities, Joyce said excitedly *"come on guys the bus is pretty empty we get the whole bus almost to ourselves. Let's get to know each other!"*

What? Girl, you ain't slick.

She was right. It was rare for the bus to be so empty at that time of the afternoon but for some reason the timing had it just so. It was only Joyce, the tall boy, me, and a couple of single moms with small kids on the bus. The weather was warm, and the bus windows were wide open. You could hear the salsa music blasting in the streets as was usually the case on a Friday afternoon in the Bronx and this seemed like it was going to be a cool ride home. And that it was.

The three of us decided to sit in the back of bus. This wasn't uncommon for high school students riding the city bus – but it was nice to have the back to ourselves. Often, particularly when we were riding with Margarita and Joyce's crew, we would sit in the back and laugh and joke and talk about the day we just had in school. A lot of the girls would be talking about people ...gossiping and carrying on.

But this day was quieter. Much. Almost serene. As the spring air wafted through the back of the bus Joyce, me and the tall boy talked about everything... and nothing at all. I don't really remember much about the conversation except to say that the conversation was fun. It felt strangely safe. I felt like I was in the company of two people who would be in my life for years to come. I was right.

We got off the bus at our third connection, and I was almost startled when the tall boy got off with us - - but then I remembered the day that he, Joyce, Margarita, and me had all gotten off the bus together that day. *"That's right,"* I thought... he lives near us. I thought back to that day in March and remembered Margarita's peculiar (and hilarious) introduction - - with all that giggling.

As we walked across the street towards the bus stop, I noticed Joyce walking very quickly ahead of us. She was so obvious. But what was she up to? Was she giving us time alone? *Don't read into it, Gigi, I thought.* Please don't be any weirder than you already are I told myself.

As we crossed the street, I did indeed notice an awkward silence between us. Finally, he broke the ice. He knew that I had a math teacher that taught him the previous year, so he asked me about my experience with her. I told him about it, and I also told him how terrible I was in math. He laughed and said that he could relate but he offered to help me because he had gotten better.

Cute. That was nice.

By this time, we had caught up with Joyce and the three of us were standing together again waiting for our last bus home. Joyce said, "Hey guys, do we just wanna walk it? " Honestly, because I lived so much further than either of them, I absolutely did NOT want to do the long walk. I was tired and it had gotten warmer still, but I was a teenager enslaved to peer pressure... *anddddd*, if I'm honest, I wasn't quite ready for the afternoon to be done - - so I agreed. "*Sure!*" I said, all over-enthusiastic and fake.

"*We can walk. A walk might be nice.*" I lied.

But surprisingly as we began our late afternoon stroll, it *was* very nice. It was June in that spring fever kind of way, and something was in the air. The tall boy and Joyce walked ahead of me. I was a slow walker, but I was close enough to them so that the three of us were having a constant banter the whole way. The tall boy had excellent vocabulary and his humor was dry and witty. He's a great conversationalist, I thought. *Hmmm.* That's nice too.

About 15 minutes into the walk, we reached the corner of the tall boy's building. As we stood on the corner ramping up to say goodbyes things became strange and clumsy. Suddenly, Joyce got quiet, then I got quiet and then the tall Black boy, DEFINITELY became quiet.

Finally, I said, *"Well Joyce, we better get going because you know how my Dad is and we have another 15 minutes because I live the furthest."*

Now, something you should understand about Black and Latin Bronx high school students in the Bronx in 1982 is that we were *very* affectionate. Particularly if you had Latine/Latina/Latino/Latinx friends, you could expect at all times to give and receive kisses hello and goodbye. That was just how we did it - - it was a part of our culture. It was very much a part of how we greeted each other. We kissed each other hello, we kissed each other goodbye and generally there was lots of physical signs of love. So, it didn't surprise me not in the least when the tall boy, who admittedly I did not know very well, leaned down to first kiss Joyce goodbye. And then he bent down to do the same with me. But because the moment was so bizarre, he moved his head in such a way to kiss me on my cheek, and I moved my head in such a way to kiss *him* on his cheek, but we were both nervous and went the wrong way and accidentally caught each other face-to-face and half kissed on the lips!

He was stunned.

But no more so than I.

Joyce audibly gasped.

Wait!??!?! What? What just happened?!?!

The three of us stood there for what was probably just 60 seconds or so, (but you know, the kind of 60 seconds that felt like eight minutes). We stood on that corner and just stared at each other. Finally, crazy Joyce burst out laughing, *"you guys are so funny… Why don't you just admit that you like each other!!"*

Was she high?

First of all, why was she saying this *in front of him*? Did she not see the ground opening up to swallow me in? Secondly, who said I liked him?!? Who said?!?

The tall boy laughed loud, nervously – and a lot.

I matched his nervous laugh, but I was NOT amused. I was embarrassed.

Then something snapped. Interestingly our tall boy became   quite   confident.

He looked directly in my eyes and said, "Wellllll... *since Joyce thinks we like each other, maybe we should exchange phone numbers?"*

Good Lord. Here we go.

I had been in this predicament before. Where a boy wanted, or maybe I volunteered, my phone number when I knew *full well* that Frankie would murder me! He had a rule, remember? No boys until we were 16. While I was going to be 15 that coming fall, I was still **not** 16, and I was only 14. If I gave the tall boy my phone number I thought, surely, he's going to call. *What would I do with Frankie?* He was going to break my neck.

I told you already that we had been through a number of hijinks in grammar school with me and little boys and me giving way my phone number, so I really didn't want to tick my Dad off again. I know that me and my pre-mature love life was fully wearing on his patience.

Oh, but this.

This sweet afternoon, in the warm spring sun, with the bud of new love, from a tall handsome older high school boy?

Oh, me and Frankie, yet again, were just going to have to fight.

I tried to play it off and pretend that I didn't care. I shrugged and said "sure, you can have my phone number." He smiled wide.

He then reached inside his knapsack and ripped off a piece of paper out of a notebook. He handed me the slip of paper and a pen, and he was like, "here write your number on here." Simultaneously, he asked Joyce to turn around and on the piece of paper he tore for himself, on the back of her back, he wrote his phone for me. *Here you go Gigi, here's my phone number. Call me anytime.*

My God, I have this teenage boy's phone number.

We said our final goodbyes, gave each other another round of hugs - - this time much more careful and calculated so that we wouldn't have any more mishaps, and Joyce and I took our leave. When we were safely out of earshot and more than a block away, Joyce let out the loudest giggle. In the most excited and enthusiastic best friend squeal, she exclaimed "*You like him! You like him! We knew it!*"

"*Who is we, Joyce?*" I was annoyed.

"We, silly, is me and Margarita. You remember that day that we rode home and all four of us got off the bus?"

"*I remember,*" I said. I hated being embarrassed.

"*Well, Margarita called me later and asked, 'do you think Gigi likes our friend? Gi, he was already asking about you back then!*"

And even though all the weirdness was starting to make sense, still, this news knocked me over.

Sort of like being at the beach waist high in the water, on the edge of the ocean when you have no intention to go all the way fully in. You're minding your business digging your toes in the cold sand under the water and enjoying the sun and all of a sudden, a huge wave comes out of nowhere, knocks you down in the sand and you have a mouth full of salty ocean water. Shocking.

Wait, what?!? He likes me? What are we talking about? How did this happen? WHEN did this happen?

We had barely had three or four conversations, and I wasn't entirely sure where all of this was coming from. But as Joyce and I walked home, and in the time that it took us to walk away from the tall boy to my house, the idea began to grow on me. Honestly, I think I more liked that someone liked me, but the thoughts came rapidly.

He *is* funny I thought.

He seems really smart; I mean he understands that crazy math and he does have a great vocabulary. And he is really tall!

When we got to Joyce's house and I kissed her goodbye, she said with smug best friend knowledge, *"you're thinking about him aren't you? You like him, don't you? Hahaahaha, Cupcake you like him."*

What on earth was she talking about it?!? I barely knew this kid. "Joyce, I've had like maybe three conversations with him. I don't know him, and he doesn't know me!" I don't think Joyce believed a word I said. She replied, *"Then why do you have that stupid smile on your face, Gigi?"* She was laughing as she went in the house singing *"Gigi likes a boyyyyyy… Gigi likes a boyyyyy."*

Oh brother. We were so young.

The budding of new love is a mystery.

It has its own velocity, and it makes up its own tempo as it goes along. In the time that it took me to walk from Joyce's house to my own, a cool quick seven-minutes maybe, a short documentary movie began to play in my mind. In those seven minutes I played back every hello in the high school hallway and every interaction I had previously had with the tall boy. All of a sudden, I remembered every time I bumped into him in the school cafeteria.

Like pressing rewind on your favorite episode, or while watching a movie, frames appeared in my mind of our hellos and chats and things started began to click. I remembered random times that I saw him on the bus in the morning and remembered seeing a slight smile. Then there was the time that I bumped into him in our high school library, and he asked if I liked to read.

It was a custom in our high school that if you had a birthday your friends would decorate your locker. On Margarita's birthday, Joyce asked me to help her decorate Margarita's locker. Once we were done, Joyce, Margarita, a bunch of their friends… AND the tall boy, gathered around Margarita's locker to sing her 'Happy Birthday.' I had forgotten that the tall boy was staring at me the entire time that morning. I wasn't paying him much attention and had just put it together moments ago after our awkward, accidental, weird half kiss on the cheek/ half kiss on the lips fiasco.

He *does* like me I thought!

Hmmm…well, whattya know!

(WHY had I never seen any of this before, I wondered.)

I don't know that in that seven-minute walk I made the decision that I liked him. I do know that I was intrigued by the idea that *he liked me*. As I reached the front gate of my parents' house, another wave hit me. This one was of schoolgirl excitement, delight, and nervousness... *And were those butterflies?* The idea was growing on me.

As I fumbled for my house keys, I found myself reliving that moment when we left the tall boy on his corner. How come that happened, I wondered? Did he mean to kiss me? Did I mean to kiss him? Why are my palms so sweaty?

Why can I find my keys?

WHAT IS HAPPENING TO ME???!?

I eventually got it together and got in the house.

It was a Friday, so unlike most days I didn't have to follow our strict afterschool routine of taking off and hanging up my uniform and getting right to my homework. I did change into my afternoon house clothes and was about to sit down and watch television when the phone rang.

"*Hello?*"

"Hi. Do you know who this is?"

Why was my heart beating like that?

"I think so. But I *just* left you."

I didn't have a lot of experience with high school boys, but I knew for sure that I said that with a ton of feminine energy - - I could HEAR my fool self, smiling. *Was I flirting*? My word.

In his next few words, I could hear him smiling back.

"Yup, that's true we just left each other but I can't stop thinking about you. What was that, Gigi? That weird thing that happened when we kissed goodbye?"

"I'm not sure. I... I..."

Lord, ... I was stuttering. "I mean, I meant to just do the normal thing, ... You know, like kiss you goodbye on the cheek all regular. And I kind of think you meant to kiss me goodbye on the cheek too... But errrr... something else happened."

"I'll say. You do know I like you right?"

"But how?" I asked. "You barely know me... We've only spoken a few times and we've only been on the bus together with those guys I think like twice. How could you like me?"

"Well, I don't want you to think I'm weird, because it's not like I've been stalking you or anything..."

We both laughed.

"But I have been watching you. You're different than the other girls. You're an outsider, like me. I know you're friendly, but you're also kind of quiet too. And I think you're pretty... really pretty."

Hi, Jesus? It's Gigi. You got a sec? Are you hearing this?

Is this happening? Are you and God punking me? Does this high school boy like me?

What on earth is happening?

I promise you that I remember this day as clearly as looking out of a freshly washed windshield.

It was June 17, 1982.

I had no idea that the rest of my life, and certainly the next 10 years, were about to drastically change.

Who knew that very afternoon I had encountered my very first love?

Certainly, in that first very tender, very innocent high school phone call I had no idea what was to come. But my life in so many ways was about to change.

"So… I guess you want to know if I like you too, huh?"

Oh sure, I was indeed flirting. I was catching on.

He chuckled.

"*Well…*" More chuckling, "I would be lying if I said I didn't think about it"

"Well, it's interesting, because I just told Joyce that I didn't know you very well."

"Oh. So… you talked to Joyce about me?"

Oh, I could really hear him smiling now.

"I did. I told her that I wasn't sure if I liked you back because we don't know each other very well. I mean I've seen you around… in the cafeteria and everything... And there was that time in the library when you asked me about books and reading... And yeah, the couple of times we were on the bus together... But honestly I don't really know you."

"Well, he said we will just have to fix that."

Ok, *he* was flirting now. I like this I thought.

"Well, I should tell you something. My parents are really, really strict. I'm really not supposed to even be talking the boys and my father has this really stupid rule that I can't have a boyfriend until I am 16."

"Oh, so you *have* thought about me being your boyfriend?"

I thought my cheeks were going to burst right off of my face, I smiling so hard.

"I don't know that I thought about it. I just found out that this might be a thing between us when I tried to give you just a friendship kiss goodbye and it turned into something else."

"Well, I guess were going to just have to see what this can turn into. I know it's the summertime and school is out for the summer, but maybe we can talk on the phone and get to know each other."

I told the tall boy that I would really like that.

And from that day, and every day through that summer, we spoke on the phone for hours each day. On Saturdays we spoke several times a day. We talked about our families, our dreams, our friends, our fears, our goals in life, We also talked about what we would do if we had a lot of money, what we would do if we had no money, we talked about God, we talked about church, we talked about school, we talked about food, we talked about death, we talked about life, and we talked about what it means to fall in love.

On that Friday, I did mention to him that I had to go back to school that following Tuesday to pick up some things from my locker and to turn in one last assignment to our Social Studies teacher.

The tall boy told me that "ironically" (yeah, right) that he too had to go into school that following Tuesday to clean out *his* locker and see a teacher. He asked me what time I was going. Classes were over and there were only a few teachers in the building doing administrative things and some students who had to do exactly what I had to do. There was no set time since classes were over. I told the tall boy that I was planning on being at the school at 11 AM or so. He told me in return that he could easily go at that time and wanted to know if I wanted to have lunch and come home together on the bus.

I told him I would like that.

That weekend was the longest of my life. Although we spoke every day on the phone that weekend the prospect of seeing him again and really trying to figure out if I did like him, or not, had me wound-up throughout that weekend. I barely slept. When Tuesday came, we had agreed that we would meet by the brass doors, go to our respective lockers, take care of our respective business, and would meet back by the brass doors in about an hour. When I arrived at the school that morning there he was with a small bouquet of flowers in his hand.

Here you go Gigi. "These are for you."

No one had EVER bought me flowers before.

"Why? It's not my birthday"

"I just wanted you to know that I think you're special."

Was there NO way to get Jesus on the phone immediately?

We were done with our end of year activities, and back at the brass doors talking about what we wanted to eat. Like I said, Bronx high school kids in those days loved pizza so that's what we decided to do. It was another warm June day and walking together was really nice. We continued our conversation and got to know each other. We got on the bus and sat next to each other and there was more than one occasion that I could feel him brushing his hand against mine. He wasn't bold enough to reach out to hold it, but I could tell he wanted to.

We ate lunch together and like a little lady I was embarrassed because I didn't want the cheese and the sauce to run down my chin. I was trying to be very ladylike as I ate in front of him.

I remember going to the counter and asking the pizza guy for a plastic knife and fork.

The tallboy cracked up when I came back to the table.

He said, "Gigi what are you doing with a knife and fork?!," as he chuckled.

"Oh, I don't know I just didn't want to get messy."

Silly girl.

It was the beginning of the purest kind of love. We were young, inexperienced, and fumbling around in it all. It was very, very sweet. After spending the day together that day there was no doubt in my mind.

Not only did I like him, but I also liked him _a lot_.

He was really very tall. At the time he was 6'3 and he believed that he wasn't finished growing! His skin was a dark chocolate brown and he had big round brown eyes. He wasn't muscular or anything… in fact he was tall and lanky; straight up and down, like the basketball guys. We talked about why he didn't play basketball in high school because he certainly had the height.

Midsummer, somewhere near August we started talking about how we couldn't wait for the school year to begin so we can see each other again.

"Do we really have to wait Gigi? Can't I come visit you?"

"I already told you that my parents are super strict. You can come and see me if you want to take your life into your own hands. My Dad is not fooling around with this rule."

"But you will be 15 in October."

"Yeah, but 15 is not 16, and my Dad won't budge on this."

For the next several days this boy continued to ask me about the possibility of him coming to visit me. He wanted to know what it would take, and I really didn't have an answer and I did not have the constitution to fight with Frankie.

Frankie was a military guy and there were many things that he had decided when he got married and had children. And one of those things, when he saw that my mom gave him girls, was that he would use every bit of his military training to break the neck of the first boy that came near us.

And he had made himself very clear over the course of our lives, that he intended to keep that promise.

No boys. Ever.

No calls from boys. No visits from boys.

No boys.

I was four years older than my little sister and as I told you, my older sister wasn't living with us, so that meant that the first-person Frankie could experiment his rules on - - was me.

I had already proven to him in my grammar school days that I had an appetite for boys. Frankie knew me well and he spoke fluent Gigi.

He wasn't having any more of my shenanigans and he watched me like a hawk!

But different than any middle school crush this high school love was big business.

This boy bought me flowers and was *pursuing me.*

Calling daily and asking to come and visit and thangs. This warranted some super big girl mature courage. I'm not sure how it happened, but I gathered it up.

One day that summer, when I gauged that Frankie was in a good mood, I said the following:

"Hey, Dad I wanted to run something by you. What if I told you that I had a new...*uhmmmm*... friend?"

He was sitting at the table reading The NY Post with a couple coffee and a cigarette and initially he wasn't paying much attention. He responded to me without looking up from the paper.

When I saw that I didn't quite have his attention, I made the decision to push further. "*Yeah, so Dad... this friend is a guy friend.*"

Slowly my father doubled-tapped his cigarette in the ashtray as he looked up at me.

"What you mean ...*a guy friend?*" His voice was stern and ready to pounce boy...lol.

"Yeah, so like at the end of the school year, I made a new friend. He was a sophomore and now he's going to be a junior and he is really nice and he's supersmart and he's been a good friend. We've been getting to know each other." I was rambling off the tall boy's credentials like a boyfriend resume.

Oh, I had his attention now.

"What you mean "you've been getting to know each other? School is out. What kind of 'getting to know' have you been doing this summer? What the hell does THAT mean?"

Easy girl. Don't blow it.

"Well… we've been talking a lot on the phone."

Brace. Brace. Brace…

Silence, but Frankie was glaring at me.

"You've been talking to him a lot on the phone. Now, is that right? Oh really. Did I give you permission for any of that?"

I could feel my father's agitation begin to rise. This wasn't going to be easy.

"Now Dad I know what your rules are. I know that I can't have a *boyfriend*. I get it. But he's not my boyfriend. He's a really cool guy who seems to come from a really good family and we like talking to each other."

I was straight lying.

Although his eyebrow was arched so high it was touching his hairline, he said "go on."

"What I was thinking was… what if, say… you met my new friend. What if you even talked to his parents on the phone? What if we made some special arrangement where he could visit under your watchful eye – the whole time."

Now between ya'll and me this was NOT exactly the arrangement I wanted.

I was pretty sure that my new gentleman caller was going to want to hold hands or kiss me …or something. At least I was hoping that!

But one step at a time.

Ya boy Frankie barked back… "Lemme think about it."

Okay! Okay! NOT a definitive 'NO' – we're in there.

I was cheesin' from ear to ear.

He did NOT like the prospect, but he was warming up to it. Walking away from me he shot back, "…and Gigi, ask me nothing about this. If, (*and I do mean IF*), I agree to this, I will let *you* know. Not another word. Let me think about. Do NOT bug me about this – you hear?"
Fair.

"You got it Dad," I won't bug you.

I planned to follow-up the next day. My mother talked me out of that bad idea and saved me from myself.

At her advice, I waited until Frankie came back to me and it wasn't long after. About a week later we were in the kitchen one morning and he turned me quite unexpectedly and said…

"Okay Miss Missy… here are the instructions for how this is going to go."
Whattttt???!?! This might happen?

"Sure Dad, whatever you say I'll do…"

Next Saturday all your Uncles will be here. Stanley, Arthur, Ernie, Dan, your Uncle Bobby… everyone. I told your mother I wanted to have the guys over for some gospel singing and a few beers."

Ugh, … I know you wanna judge, but we're a complicated family. Beers and singing about Jesus went hand in hand. Hard to explain. Stay with me.

This is how they spent time together. Singing hymns and drinking liquor. Whatcha gon' do?

"Tell your little friend," ('little friend' said with disgust and disdain), "that he can come over from 1pm to 8pm but before he visits with _you_, I need to have a man-to-man with him. Got it?"

Gulp. Got it.

So, I asked Frankie, "Will he have to face the uncles as well?"

I mean I cared for the boy, quite the bit, the last thing I was trying to do was set him up.

"We'll cross that bridge when we get to it." Frankie said. That was just going to have to be enough for me.

My father did go on to say though that he was requiring a phone call between himself and the father of my new "little friend."

Very, very cool.

But as Frankie walked away from me, he gave me a look that said "step out of line just ONE-time little girl and I will break your neck and you will be 90-years old before the next time you see the inside of a date. "

I got it, for real this time.

I got on the phone with my "little friend," and I told him the good news. "What?! What? … I can come and see you?"

Easy partna.

I explained to my friend, "Well…we have some steps we gotta follow. First, my Dad wants to speak to your Dad. Can we do that? "

He said sure and he didn't think that was going to be a problem.

And then I will warn you, part of the reason that I think that he's okay with you coming over next Saturday is because all my uncles will be here-all of them.

"Will I have to meet them to?"

"I'm not sure, but if I were you, I would be ready for like a panel discussion."

"A what? A panel discussion?!"

"No silly, but actually. *Wellll*, honestly, I'm not sure. Maybe. Like, kinda. Be prepared."
We cracked up.

"Just know this, there will be a number of southern Black men here in our house that Saturday who are going to want to talk to you. Just be yourself and make it plain that you have no intention to hurt me, and I think we'll get through it."

My friend said in the sweetest teenage way possible,

"Well, #1, I would never hurt you, and #2 Gigi I think you're worth it, so I can't wait."

Swoon.

The following Saturday couldn't come fast enough. While I knew it was going to be a grueling hazing session for my friend, I'm still just a girl. I liked him so much by this point, and I wanted to look nice. I picked out a really nice pair of jean pants and I asked my mom for $20 so that I could go to Alexander's and buy a new shirt.

I was 14 and I didn't wear makeup, but I called my older sister Trease and told her what was happening. I asked her what I should do.

She said, "well just make sure you wear lip gloss...and don't smile too much. Wear the lip-gloss though because he might want to kiss you."

Oh Lord, I hope so! I also liked having a big sister.

The day came and my new friend called at around 12:30 PM. He said I'm on my way is it still, okay?

All early.

I understood why he asked because we were both not sure if Frankie was going to change his mind. But I told him that it was still okay and that my family was looking forward to meeting him.

At PROMPTLY 12:50 the doorbell rang, and it was him.

He had on a pair of Black slacks, nice Black shoes, a light blue polo shirt and a sweater vest. The one thing about my friend and I was that we were pretty much both corn balls. He was nerdy-just like me.

Sweater vests where appropriate.

It was the first time we had seen each other since the day we met at school, and it was great to see him. We hugged nervously and awkwardly, and we did so on the front porch.

I told him, "come on in, let's get this over with."

I also asked if he felt okay, and he told me that he was really very nervous.
Well of course you are! My father was terrifying.

When he came into the living room Frankie was standing not far behind me in the kitchen.

I was so proud of my new friend.

Without hesitation, he stuck his hand out like a man and said,

"Good afternoon Mr. Gilliard, is so good to meet you in person. It was nice talking to you on the phone earlier this week and I'm glad you had a chance to talk to my father. Thank you for having me in your home."

My new friend had in his hands two flower bouquets: one was slightly larger than the other. The larger bouquet was for my mother and instead of taking it upon himself to simply hand the bouquet to her, he asked my Dad,

"Mr. Gilliard these flowers are for your wife. Would it be okay if I presented her with these?" Obviously, he had been coached. No 15-year-old was that mature.

Now y'all you HAVE to know that in this very moment, even at 14, I simply knew for sure that I was going to marry this boy. FOR.SURE.

My father said in response to my new friend, "Welcome son, very nice gesture of flowers for my wife, and flowers for my Gigi. You'll get some brownie points for that."

My friend looked down and laughed, and Frankie laughed with him. It was the beginning of their friendship. My friend went into the kitchen and did indeed meet my Mom, presented her with the flowers and then he met Gida. Uh boy.

And no matter how hard we tried that relationship just never worked. We should have all known from the very first meeting.

"You must be the little sister," he said.

Gida studied him for a few minutes. She looked him up and down disapprovingly... like "who is this guy?"

She was 10 years old, nearly 11 herself, and not quite as fast as I with boys, and thus, not exactly sure what to do with him.

"No dummy, I'm the Mom... Of course, I'm the little sister. You my sister's boyfriend?" We all laughed because everybody knew that none of us were supposed to be talking about that.

Mom offered my friend something to eat and a glass of Kool-Aid. He was super polite and thanked her. He said he wasn't hungry, but he was thirsty. Mom poured him some Kool-Aid, and she's suggested that he go on downstairs and meet my Dad in the basement. She showed him where to go and down into the abyss he went.

Oh boy, here we go.

Interestingly, I noticed that all my uncles were in the backyard. They had already started singing their gospel with Uncle Stanley leading them and I think they were already doing a little drinking too.

When I peeked out the back door I realized, oh Dad and my friend are in the basement alone. Oh dear.

I wasn't sure whether to be happy about that or more concerned. But I did think at least he didn't have to face the Council of uncles like I thought Dad was going to make him do.

They might've been downstairs for I don't know, 30 minutes maybe? It felt like hours.

Finally, they emerged.

When the basement door opened all we heard was more laughter. The laughter I heard from my friend was that of relief, you know after a big test or after you you kill it in a big presentation.

I heard in his voice the sound of "*whew!*"

When they came upstairs, Dad said to him, "Mr. Young Man, your parents raised you well. I appreciate you being a man about our talk today, but I will need you to remember everything I told you in the basement, you understand?"

From that moment that's how Frankie referred to him, as Mr. Young Man. For the next nearly ten years Frankie greeted him regularly with, "Well, hello Mr. Young Man," or "how are you Mr. Young Man," "Nice to see you again Mr. Young Man."

Seldom did I hear my Dad use his name, but Mr. Young Man stuck and had come to make sense.

As young romances go, we were off to the races.

That afternoon after the basement talk, Mr. Young Man and I sat on the front step, and we laughed and drank Kool-Aid. He did kiss me… ever so carefully and I could tell that my father had given him a serious talking to.

That afternoon would mark the beginning of many, many Saturday afternoons together over the next decade. Mr. Young Man and I dated all through high school, and then all through college, and then for a couple of years beyond that.

After his basement meeting with my Dad, we went back to high school the following year feeling like we had permission to take our relationship public. On the first day of school, he called to arrange to meet Joyce and I so that the three of us could take the bus together. When we got on the bus, I sat in between he and Joyce.

This time he took my hand proudly, and Joyce and I giggled about it.

As we got off the bus, we were still holding hands and we boldly walked into school like a proud boyfriend and girlfriend big time high school couple.

118

As we came past the bronze doors that marked the main school entrance, one of the first people we saw in the hallway was Jeanine.

I've shared so much with you about Joyce, but Jeanine was also my childhood best friend. In fact, I've known Jeanine longer than any other friend I've had. Jeanine's family and mine attended the same church in Harlem. We had known each other since we were very little girls in Sunday school at church. We met when we were about eight (although we sometimes argue about this now because we can't remember if we were seven or eight... but suffice it to say we've been friends for a lifetime).

We participated in Sunday school pageants, Christmas shows, and even sang on the church choir together for a brief time. When we got to orientation day at high school during our first year the year previous... Jeanine said, "What are _you_ doing here?! I only see you at church!"

I retorted, "What are _you_ doing here?!" And from that moment on we were thrilled, and convinced, that our friendship had been destined.

Jeanine was and is very Black. Most of the people she hung around with in high school were the Black girls and she was a member of the African American club. Because Frankie insisted that I come straight home after school, my club involvement in high school was severely limited. That made Jeanine my bridge to the Black world in high school. Our high school had a very small Black population. So having a connection to the high school Black community and was important, particularly for girl like me who spent a lot of time with my Latina friend. Jeanine was my bridge to that world.

Not only was Jeanine my bridge to my Black friends in high school, but she was also my fiercest protector. Fierce is probably the first word that comes to the minds of most when you meet her.

Jeanine is a beautiful, bold, direct, confident, no nonsense, all female energy, and one of the fiercest protector-friends around. She knew Mr. Young Man very well. In part because of his own connection to the African American club in the 'Black kids' circle they both ran in. And she did NOT like him very much,

Jeanine will tell you openly, to this day, that she was never fond of me and Mr. Young Man hanging out together. Not even a little bit. I don't know that she trusted him, or his friends and she never wanted me to get hurt.

As we ran into Jeanine on the morning of the first day of my sophomore year – his Junior – the day I was making my relationship with Mr. Young Man public – Jeanine's disgust was apparent. She said nothing.

I was literally giddy with excitement and Mr. Young Man was walking very confidently with his new little girlfriend. When she saw us, her right eyebrow raised in an arch (the way a cat's back is prone to do before an attack). Yeah. Jeanine couldn't stand this kid and her eyebrow raise is notorious.

Well, when you are a girl like me, warnings about getting hurt from your best friend are easy to pooh-

pooh. I assured Jeanine that Mr. Young Man had the best intentions and that he was a good guy.

Her response to me was another dangerously raised eyebrow.

Organically though, Mr. Young Man and I became a well-known high school item in the mid-80s. People started to address us, *as an us*. We were far more mature for our age and over the years we both surmised that because we came from families that saw very little divorce, coupling was the norm for us. We OFTEN gave advice to other teenage couples and even held "counseling sessions" with the school cafeteria with couple who were bickering. It was not uncommon for us to bump into one another during a change of class and me hear "Babe, Arthur and Lilly are really having trouble. Can we sit them at lunch and help them work on their friendship?" No joke.

We were outrageous!

Additionally, we were both quite tied to the Latin community. We both had best friends and deep relationships with people who identified as Latin/Latine/Latina/Latinx.

Many of our Latin friends, even those who began dating as teenagers, stayed together until marriage. Interestingly enough, as Bronx Black kids we were influenced by that. We both saw a lot of marriage in our family. It stood to reason that we would be influenced by that. Even as kids, we talk a lot about what it would mean to get married after high school.

Now, neither one of us thought that marriage _right_ after high school was a great idea, but certainly staying together and marrying your high school sweetheart was a consistent topic of conversation all the time.

As we moved through high school years, we were experiencing life together. We saw people die in our families, we saw various family dynamics play out around us, we experienced more than one high school friend pass away, we were making plans for college - - we were growing up together.

Mr. Young Man being one year ahead of me meant that he graduated high school and went on to college the whole year before I did. We talked about me coming to his college and he encouraged me to apply in my senior year.

Frankie had been very generous allowing me and Mr. Young Man to begin dating before I was 16, allowing Mr. Young Man to come over frequently for long visits, really making this a young man a part of our lives if I'm honest.

But my Pops drew the line about me going to the same college with this boy.

Nope. THAT was *NOT* happening.

He said, "Girl, you must think I'm crazy... Do you honestly think I would allow you to be alone on the same campus with this boy that you been in love with for the last almost four years? No ma'am, you can pick any school you can get into, but you CANNOT go to college with him."

He liked Mr. Young Man well enough, but my father was still a man - - who understood teenage boys.

"Forget it Sista."

Oddly, while I was mildly disappointed, I got it.

I knew for certain that I wouldn't focus, and I thought for sure that I would be a distraction to Mr. Young Man as well. But he was going to school on Long Island, and I made the best decision to attend Rutgers: the State University of New Jersey which meant that we were only a two-hour train ride away from one another, at worst.

But by the time Mr. Young Man became a senior in college I could feel that the strain of the distance... Even the distance of a two-hour train ride was too much for our childhood romance.

Mr. Young Man had discovered other girls, other interests, and he was growing up and growing *away* from me. I too was interested in new things, and learning myself, and thinking about my future.

But never in a million years did my future ever <u>not</u> include Mr. Young Man.

After we had both graduated, and after we had already started to drift apart, those last two years of our relationship were quite rocky. Jeanine spent a lot of time consoling me on the phone in those days and one afternoon she said to me:

"Gi, I think you need to face it. You guys have grown apart." I fought her saying, "you've never liked him so you're not willing to imagine that we might make it." "No Gi, I could just always see that he wasn't your forever dude. I always saw that."

It was hard to hear her, but Jeanine always kept things 100% real. She loved me greatly and could see that Mr. Young Man wasn't nearly as attentive as he once had been when we were kids. He wasn't nearly as enamored with me as the 15-year-old charming young boy coming to visit his first girlfriend.

Indeed, we had drifted well apart.

Not long after graduating college, Mr. Young Man got an apartment with some of his college buddies. No longer did he need to ask Mr. Gilliard permission to come and see me at the house - - because we spent a lot of "grown up time" at his place.

One night, as I planned to stay over, he said to me

"Gi, we should make a pact."

This was curious.

"What kind of a pact?," I asked.

He said, "I think we should agree that if we don't make it, if our relationship doesn't stand the test of time, I think we should agree that if we go on to marry other people in the future, we won't ever stay in touch with each other."

What? What was he talking about?

First, why are we thinking about not making it?
And why so dramatic?

When I look back on it now surely this was his way to begin the uncoupling. He was setting the stage. Conditioning my mind for what was to come. I protested and said I don't know why we are thinking about this, but okay if we don't make it and we end up breaking up, we will stay away from each other.

I was dumbfounded. Where was this coming from?

His rationale was that the intense love of high school sweethearts who had been in a long-term relationship- - love between two people who grew up together sharing as much as we had in our formative years - - would be hard to let go of. He thought it would be hard to resist one another in the future if we were both in relationships with new people and he wanted to be faithful in a new relationship.

I didn't buy it. It sounded like somebody who wanted to break up to me - - and wanted it to be a clean break at that. I told him so and he said I wasn't being fair.

My heart was breaking, fair wasn't on the table.

Later that evening, as I sat on the side of his bed, he continued to behave strangely.

He asked, "you know what I've never done?"

"No, what?"

He said, "I've never set your hair in rollers." I cracked up. "What?!" This was nuts.

Why would you want to do that, I asked? Did he want to practice for the next girl?

I was super suspicious now, but real talk I had always known him to be tremendously nostalgic and highly sentimental. It was one of things that drew me to him those years ago as young teens.

He explained that it was just something that he had always wanted to do and had never asked.

"I've always wanted to experience what it was like to roll up your hair and I don't want us to part without out doing that." Oh, so we're parting. Oh my.

Okay, sir. This was bizarre.

My hair was much longer and much thicker then. You probably won't find many Black women who still use pink sponge rollers now, but back then I used them all the time.

Still suspect, I acquiesced.

In the most interesting, yet tender and very sad way, I taught Mr. Young Man on our last night together how to roll up my hair. He put on a mixed tape of our favorite love songs, and he rolled up my hair while we both cried. He stopped a few times and leaned into the back of my head and whispered, "I'll never stop loving you, Gigi. I mean that."

Other than that, neither of us spoke except for me to give him gentle instructions on how to make the parts straight so he could make even rows for the rollers. By this time, we both knew that our time together had come to an end.

Naturally, there was more drama and some more tears over the coming weeks, but on the night of the pink roller set, we did indeed say goodbye.

The next day I stayed in bed and wept all day.

I called my older sister, I called Jeanine, and I called Joyce.

Up until that time in my life I had never known a pain like that one.

I believed that grief was only for death.

I never understood that the ending of relationships, and the painful churn of a major life transition could bring such deep and hollow sorrow.

Outside of all that were the ways that I began to feel insecure about myself; all the questions that obsessed my mind for the next several months: was I not pretty enough? Was I too fat (we had talked a lot about the weight I had gained in my later high school years, weight that I never really lost)? Maybe I just wasn't good enough. I didn't understand that the ending of a relationship could bring such a complete feeling of loss. I lost a sense of security, a sense of connection - - and I had certainly lost a sense of myself. We had been together for so long through those formative years that the ending of this relationship brought to me a trauma previously unknown.

I would only come to see Mr. Young Man once more.

But aside from that time, up until the time of his death, we kept our pact.
In the days of social media, he found me, and we connected briefly.

Neither one of us saying not one word to the other - - but he could see me online… and I could see him, but we did indeed kept far away from one another,

Literally... *for the rest of our lives.*

Well, hello heartbreak.

Chapter 4

Dungeons & Dragons

G"igi,"

I could hear a strain in his voice, what was this about I wondered?

"We need you to come home."

"What's going on Dad, why do you need me to come home?"

I had only heard this kind of urgency mixed with the intense sound of sadness in my father's voice when there was a death in the family.

"Can I just get you to come home please... I want to share with you some things when you get here."

I hated when he was like this.

I wasn't going to be able to leave where I was right away, so wasn't going to be able to get home until hours later. I was wishing that he would just come out and say what was happening while we were on the phone.

But he did not.

I got home, and sure enough Mom was crying, and so was he. I've mentioned to you a couple of times that I lived for a short while with my Cousin Janie and Susie, their Dad, and siblings, when their Mom, (my Grand aunt, Aunt Neat), was my caretaker as a little girl.

This meant that Janie and Susie and their three brothers Bobby, Cousin Boobie, and Cousin Jimmy were like older siblings as well. When I got home that day, Dad said that Cousin Boobie had passed away.

Dad himself had gone down to Harlem to see about the situation and to help my Cousins through this ordeal. We were all heartbroken and my cousin's death was shocking and unexpected.

This was during a time when Frankie and his own brothers and sisters were very involved in the same church out in Queens. For a long time, Frankie struggled in his faith, but he found his way and became a Deacon in his congregation. As such, it wasn't surprising when Cousin Boobie passed away that Dad was asked to participate in his service. At Cousin

Boobie's Homegoing, Dad shared a message about how we will all have to *"go this way"* one day.

He was encouraging the family and friends in attendance at the service to get to know God.

After the service and the repast, Mom asked me if I was going back to my apartment in the North Bronx.

"No," I said, "I think I'll just stay with you guys tonight."

But the truth is my old bedroom in my parents' house was on the top floor and for whatever reasons after a funeral... even after the funeral of a dear loved one, I never slept well. I think as a kid I was afraid of the dead, for sure but this was more about sadness.

I just didn't want to be alone - - even at my parents'.

So, at the risk of you judging me again, I took my pillow and my blanket, and I made a pallet in the downstairs bathroom outside of my parents' and Gida's bedroom.

I just wanted to be close to them I suppose, and I wanted to keep a light on all night, and I thought it would be easy to keep the light on in the bathroom.

That's totally weird, I know.

Naturally, somebody got up to use the bathroom in the middle of the night. That somebody happened to be Frankie. Not only was he startled, but he was greatly annoyed with me. "Gigi, what are you doing in the bathroom on the floor, with the light on?" He yelled.

"Dad, I was nervous sleeping upstairs. So, I just came down here." Frankie was not amused with me...

"And you thought it was a good idea to sleep on the bathroom floor with the light on? Girl, if you don't go to bed!"

Well, I couldn't sleep in Gida's room... and I certainly couldn't, at 24, sleep in the room with *them* - - so this was the next best thing.

I didn't like that he wasn't being insensitive, and I told him so, "Why are you yelling at me? We just had a death in the family Dad, I'm really sad and I do not want to be by myself!"

"Watch your tone, Miss Missy...I am very aware that we had a death in the family Gigi, But you're the one with all this renewed faith - - so why are you so afraid."
"I never said I was afraid! I said I was *sad*."

He was getting on my last nerves.

I sucked my teeth, loud, grabbed my blanket and my pillow, said 'forget it' in a huffed and I stomped upstairs. I was being a big baby. He called after me and told me not have an attitude, that he was just trying to help me be stronger.

I shot back, "Whatever Daddy" and I went to bed.

I had become looser with my fresh tongue with him in my mid-twenties - - but I knew not to push it.

But I *was* mad, and NOT feeling him.

Earlier that evening I had asked if he could give me a ride back uptown to my apartment the next day.

The next morning, still mad at him, "and with my butt on my shoulder" as he and Mother loved to say, I told him I didn't need a ride after all. I didn't have a car at the time so I gathered up my things and I told him never mind - - I would take the bus. He laughed at me (he knew I was still angry), and told me I was being ridiculous... He further insisted and said –

"Silly girl, I will happily take you home."

"No thanks," I said," I find my own way home."

"Suit yourself Gitchigumie, your pride will be the death of you." Gitchigumie was his pet name for me. None of us knew where he got it from, but usually I loved hearing. Right now, though, it was irritating me.

I was only a couple of years out of college and didn't have real luggage. I couldn't tell you, WHAT I had my overnight things in, but as I lifted the bag with my overnight things – the bag broke. All my toiletries, my nightgown, and the dress I'd worn to the funeral the day before - - everything spilled out all over the floor.

Ugh. That's what I get for being sassy.

Frankie was in the kitchen, but he was in ear shot of the whole thing and I could hear him stifling a laugh.

"You okay in there?" I sucked my teeth at him again, under my breath this time because although mad - - I was also embarrassed. I found a huge shopping bag in my mother's plastic bags stash, and I gathered up my things and threw them inside.

At this point, I felt like I _had_ to ask for a ride home, so with my tail between my legs I sheepishly asked, "I know I said I would get on the bus, but would you mind taking me home." *eyeroll*

He loved this moment. Like me, he could be *so petty.*

Like a little kid who was proven right, he said, "Sure, I'll take you home." Smirk.

But my father had the most endearing way of infuriating you one moment, and cracking you all the way up the next. Within moments of me climbing into his van he had me in stitches. But first, he wanted to talk about Cousin Boobie's service.

He asked me what I thought of the message he shared the day before. I told him that I thought it was appropriate and heartfelt. I also told him that I believed that Janie and Susie and Jimmy and Bobby were grateful. He said he hoped so.

He went on to share that he missed their Mom, Aunt Neat, so much and quite vulnerably said that his first cousin's death made him miss his own mother. I felt such compassion for him on that car ride as we talked.

As we continued uptown, he said to me that something about the morning of our cousin's funeral reminded him of the morning of his own Dad's funeral.

Clearly, he was feeling nostalgic and reflective.

I asked what he meant.

He said you and I always seem to have these deep talks whenever there is a death in the family.

I agreed.

And then I remember what he was referring to.

In my sophomore year at Rutgers, I had an 8 o'clock class on Monday mornings. It was some type of sociological theory course. While I loved the professor, I sometimes had trouble keeping up with the readings because the class was so early in the morning. I was undisciplined with my time and would often not do the reading in the evening the Sunday before... making it hard for me to get up before the class and get the reading done.

This one Monday, I had not done the reading and had the nerve to raise my hand during lecture to answer a question. I promptly embarrassed myself by not knowing the answer and making it plain to all that, obviously, I had not read the work. Sitting back behind me in the lecture hall were a group of smarty-pants girls who _had_ done the reading. They answered the question like Rhodes scholars, and I felt like a big loser-dummy. When class was over, I went back to my room to take a nap. Not sure why, but during this nap I had a _very_ vivid dream. Vivid to the point of it feeling like-a-movie-dream.

This is not uncommon for me I often dream quite vividly and can remember large pieces of what I've dreamt in great detail. This dreaming business has gotten me trouble.

In real life during the previous summer, I landed a summer job through a college intern program at the New York Human Resources Administration.

In my dream, I was back at that job that I held the previous summer. In the dream, I dreamt that Frankie called me at work and said, "you need to come home."

 In the dream, I asked him "why, has something happened?"

The exchange in my dream was very similar to the exchange that Frankie and I had in real life just days earlier about our cousin.

Back in the dream, when I arrived home my father told me that my grandfather, his Dad - Leroy Gilliard had had a heart attack. The dream was so real and so vivid, I woke feeling disturbed, and called home immediately.

Frankie answered the phone, and I asked, "Hey, Dad have you spoken to your father?"

"My Dad?"

"Yeah, _your_ Dad... my Grand Dad."

Franke then told me that he had spoken to his own father just a few days earlier and that my grandfather seemed fine. He asked me why asked, but I was reluctant to tell him the details of the dream. What I _did_ say was that I had had a troubling dream and that my grandfather was in the middle of it.

My Dad then asked me how often I spoke with my grandfather in real life? I admitted that I didn't speak with him often, and that I should call him more. My father agreed and went on to admonish me that I should, definitely, call my grandfather more. He then asked again if I was sure that I didn't want to share my dream with him. I was sure. I didn't want to upset him.

I told him that I didn't want to tell him, but that I would call him later in the week.

What I did do though, before I went to my next class was called my grandfather. I sensed that it best not to wait. My grandfather picked right up, and we had a wonderful exchange. First thing he wanted to know was how I was doing in school. I was still feeling so badly about the lecture hall incident that happened in the morning, so I shared with my grandfather how I insecure I felt around smart college kids, and that I didn't know if I was going to make it to graduation.

I was being dramatic. The truth was, all I needed to do *was just do the reading...* but I was feeling sorry for myself. My grandfather replied,

"Baby girl... I have one question. What is your last name?"

"What Grand Daddy?"

"You heard me girl, what is your last name?"

... This was hilarious.

I had the same last name as my grandfather and he knew that, but he wanted me to say it. I said, "Grand Daddy Leroy, I am a Gilliard." He was being smart and replied, "say what now!? I didn't hear what you said…" He wanted me to say it again. "Grand Daddy, my last name is Gilliard. I AM A GILLIARD."

"A'ight then. That's the end of that. You are a Gilliard and those college ch'urn don't have nothing better than you."

Except discipline, I thought.

He went on to say, yes you are a Gilliard, and you can do anything you want to do.

Nobody encourages you more than your grandparents, boy. And he was the last of my grandparents at that point. My Dad's Mom, my Grandma Sarah and both my Mom's parents, my Grand Daddy Aaron ("Doc") and my Grandma Mary had all passed away. Hearing my Grand Father do the "Gilliard" pep talk was a SUCH a crackup… And so very, very encouraging.

In real life - - just one month later.

My dream made sense.

Eerily, I did get a call in my dorm room at Rutgers. It was Frankie and he was, yes, asking me to come home.

In that call when I asked him what was going on, he said something happened with your Grandfather and we need you to get home.

I got on the first train back to New York from New Brunswick and by the time I had reached home I was unfortunately given the news that my dear Grand Daddy LeRoy had passed away from a heart attack.

On the morning of my Grandfather's funeral, Frankie caught me alone as we about to leave and he asked, "I know you didn't want to tell me before, but that day at school when you dreamt about my father - what was it about?"

 Quietly, almost in a whisper, I told Frankie that in my dream, my grandfather had had a heart attack and I dreamt very clearly that he, (Frankie, my Dad), had asked me to come home. He said, … *I knew it. I knew that's what you dreamt.*

He then asked if I called him like he told me to. I told him I did, and he was so happy that I had.

He wanted to know the conversation word for word. He was hurting so much, he wanted to hear his father's words. I told him that I had shared with my Grandfather that I was feeling insecure about being a college student and that Granddaddy did the "Gilliard pep talk" with me. He asked me to tell him what my last name was. Simultaneously we burst out laughing because Frankie did that "Gilliard Pep Talk" thing with me all the time where he would make me tell him my last name. I told him, Grand Daddy asked me just like you often do, what's your last name? And he insisted, that I say that I was a Gilliard out loud. We both laughed so hard. He did the same thing you do; and it was hilarious.

Frankie asked me, "Gi, where do you think I got that from?"

Of course, I thought. Of course.

So, on the car ride to my apartment on the day after our cousin's funeral I could see why he was so reminiscent of his father's passing. We had a very similar exchange on the phone where Frankie was asking me to come home. We also both remarked how real that dream was for me and how he, Frankie, always believed that God somehow showed me his father's passing in that dream – like a premonition.

"We're really connected you and me. I think God told you first that pain was coming my way."

Maybe, I said. Maybe. My dream was certainly real.

We marveled on that ride home about the way the brain works, and about how the subconscious works.

We talked more about premonitions, and spiritual things and the way God talks to us. He shared some personal things with me on that ride about how much he loved my mother.

"Where did THAT come from?" I wanted to know.

I'm not sure why he chose that moment to share that, but he told me that it was important to him that I knew that my mother was the only woman he had ever loved. I told him I knew that and asked why he was telling me that.

He said he wasn't quite sure, but it was important to him that I knew, and that he told me right then.

"And besides, Gitchigumie, you're my best friend."

It was strange and wonderful to be best friends with your Dad.

He was my Dude.

In that conversation I also told him that I had been given a lead for job in North Carolina. I told him that I wasn't entirely sure about the role, but it sounded like it might be a good fit for me. I asked him what he thought about me considering a job in North Carolina, and me moving away. And he said,

"Let me ask you a question, do you have a job now?" I told him I did not, and he knew that. I wasn't working at the time. He responded, "well, there's your answer. Go where the work is. You've never been afraid of opportunity. Go for it. Don't wait. *Never wait Gigi.*"

We got to the front of my apartment, and I was just about to get out and I asked him,

"Why do you think I'm your best friend?"

He replied,

"I don't know Gitchie, you seem to have always understood my demons - - and love me anyway."

Dad, I *do* love you - with big Gigi love.

I love you too Gi, with big Dad love.

****

That following Tuesday morning I was trying to get to Jersey City. My older sister was in Jersey City visiting her best friend and she had my niece with her. My niece LeAndra had just been born three weeks prior and Trease needed some help with the baby during the day.

Considering I wasn't working, I told her that I would be happy to get over there and to help her out.

As usual, the traffic on the Cross Bronx Expressway getting to the George Washington Bridge was a nightmare, but finally I made it to my sister and precious new baby niece. We spent the day together.

My sister told me how Dad had come to see her the previous Saturday and spent the whole day with her and the baby. She told me that he sat in the rocking chair all day and held my niece and talked and played with her for hours. Trease said that they had an amazing time together.

My older sister was thrilled that she and Dad and her baby had that time. It was so good. I was thrilled to hear it. Soon, it came time for me to leave and get back on the road back to the Bronx.

The traffic at the bridge getting back to the Bronx was far worse than that of the morning. I was listening to 1010 WINS on the radio, and they were reporting that there had been a terrible accident early that morning that had snarled Bronx traffic all day.

I thought, "Boy, I hope those folks are okay. "Finally, I made it home.

I got back to my apartment just in time as we were having a single girls Bible study that evening and I needed to prepare.

Just as I was changing my clothes to get ready for our Bible study guests, Mom called.

"Gi, can you come home."

Lord.

Here we go again, what now.

Evidently the car that had been in the accident that was reported on 1010 WINS, and had snarled Bronx traffic all day, had been my father.

Frankie had been in a very serious accident.

We needed to get to the hospital and figure out what condition he was in and what was going on. I did bother changing clothes. I just went to go meet my mother.

When we arrived at the hospital it was hard for us to get any information as he was in ICU critical care. By the time we found the attending physician we were ushered into a "family room" where we were met by my Dad's two brothers and another doctor.

The doctor explained that Dad had been in an terribly serious accident after having had a mild heart attack at the wheel of his van. Immediately following this information, they gave Mom and I an opportunity to go see him. Mom choose not to go into the room right way, so I went in to see him alone. He was attached to a number of whirring machines that were evidently helping him breathe and keeping him alive.

Frankie had been critically injured. The doctor was in the room saying something in my ear but all I could think about was car ride just days earlier. He said we were connected. I believed it.

Could I telepathically *will* him to live? Let's try it.

While the doctor droned on, I tried to use psychic powers. I felt desperate and stared at his forehead. *"Hey…hey …Dad. It's Gitchie. You need to breathe, Daddy. C'mon.* BREATHE."

Nothing. I barely heard a word the doctor said.

Mom and I left the ICU area, and we went back down to meet my uncles to discuss what needed to happen next. While my Mom was talking to my uncles, I knew that I needed to get a hold of my sisters.

All of this was long before cell phones, so I needed to walk down the hospital hall to find the bank of payphones. I spoke to my older sister who said that she was going to get off the phone, wrap up baby and get a ride with her friends over to the Bronx. She was talking a mile a minute, asking me tons of questions while admonishing me to stay calm.

She said that she was going to leave in 20 minutes. I told her okay, to be careful and that I saw Dad and I thought that everything was going to work out.

I lied.

We are back to the family waiting room, and I could see that my Mom was visibly upset and shaking. I was trying to kick into, "be-the-daughter-that-takes-charge-of-things" so I approached the administrator who was in the patient area with us.

I asked her what we needed to do next.

She, not knowing that I hadn't heard the news yet, said,

"Oh sweetie, the only thing to do now is to call the funeral home at this point."

Out of the corner of my eye, in a flash of a second, I saw my Uncle Arthur lunge towards me trying to stop the lady before she said anything more.

"Call the funeral home for who? Why?" I asked with an attitude.

Was she high?

But here it came.

The doctor who had ushered Mom and I to ICU, approached me gently and said:

"Miss Gilliard, I am so very sorry, but your father's body expired at 9:48 PM this evening."

****

This is hard to write. It's killing me, actually.

But it's vitally important that I keep going.

If I'm going to do this healing thing, and if I'm going to do this open thing, I need to tell you about this, but I'm struggling. Right in this moment.

We got back to the house that night and everything became a blur.

Our house immediately filled with relatives. Certainly, Dad's brothers and sisters were with us first, as our home was as much their home - - they had spent so much time with us there. But there were other visitors as well. Streams and streams of visitors.

And there was the constant phone ringing. About 15 minutes after we had come home from the hospital, I found a way to steal away from everyone.

I needed to talk to God.

Uncle Bob was sitting in Gida's room and talking with her – breaking the news to her. She had been at work on the other side of the Bronx when everything was happening. I think someone went to pick her up from job or something.

My older sister Trease was in my parents room with the baby, she was crying and talking to my brother and my Aunt ToTo was in there with them.

Aunt Gracie and Uncle Arthur and Uncle Dan were making calls to the family.

I was grateful for all of the raucous because I could slip down into the basement. I wasn't fond of the basement. It felt like a dungeon to me. But no more than this particular night. The basement was Frankie's hang out. He had converted it to his man cave, and it had all the things he liked. It had his big TV, and all his books and all his fish tanks.

Frankie loved fish and had raised tropical fish for years.

"Loved." Past tense. I remember that thought was the first time I began to refer to my father in the past tense.

In the back of the basement was our laundry room. And that's where I found the spot I was looking for. I needed a place to pray. I needed to get on my knees and beg God for this outrageous request I was about to make. With my face in the laundry basket, I presented a deal to God.

In my mind, I was trying to calculate how long a person could be dead before they could be revived again. I'm not sure if I was having a break in reality or if the dragon of grief was causing me to go into some type of shock - - but in my mind, I absolutely believed that if God wanted to - - He could revive Frankie right then.

He could simply have the doctors call and tell us that within the last hour, *miraculously*, they were able to revive Frankie. Or that, with great apology, they had made a terrible, terrible error and Frankie was now awake from his coma and that it was another husband, brother, brother-in-law, Deacon, Dad who had died. But not mine.

I started petitioning for this miracle. I was praying, I guess, but I was actually negotiating. I was promising God all kinds of things, and was begging… and weeping… and begging.

And trying to make a ridiculous contract with the Lord.

I asked God, with full seriousness, that when I went back upstairs and talked to Aunt Gracie, I wanted her to say that the hospital called and said it was all a mistake, and that her brother, my father, Sinobia's husband… this incredible human, was still alive. I wanted the hospital to tell my Auntie that we could come on back and talk to him and marvel in this mystery recovery.

I believed it would happen. I promise you I did.

I came upstairs and went straight for my Aunt. I saw that she was getting off the phone and I stood nearby and waited with anticipation. *Surely…*

But she was only talking to other relatives…and not the hospital. As the hours ticked on that evening and Frankie went from one our dead, to two hours dead, to three hours dead…

I knew that our lives would never be the same.

I knew that "I' would never be the same.

That Nothing.Would. Ever.Be. The.Same.

****

We planned the services, and everything and everybody was wonderful. There were a lot of cakes.

So wonderful. The chicken was tasty, the potato salad was mixed just so. The cakes were fresh, the pies were hot and there were folding chairs and iced tea for days.

Frankie would have loved all this attention.

He was a star, man.

He would've loved to have known that he packed out the place.

His wake was standing room only. People waited on a line that stretched *outside of* the funeral home coming to pay respects to this guy.

It cracks me up to think about how much he would have loved it all.

Bwhahahahahhahaha. He would have eaten it up.

As we sat on the front row during the wake, I saw and heard both my silly sisters whispering and giggling. I wondered what's the matter with these two? It wasn't until my brother said, "Hey Gi, look, ain't that your old flame?"

I turned around and sure enough, there was Mr. Young Man with his Mom and his Dad. They had come to pay their respects as well.

Mom graciously got up and greeted them, as did I, and they were wonderful.

Mr. Young Man whispered, "You good?" I replied, "I am *not* good."

He said "I need to pay my respects to your Pops. Come with me?"

"Of course," I said.

Mr. Young Man took my hand, and together we stood at Frankie's casket. Almost immediately we cracked up remembering the Saturday inquisition in the basement. I had NEVER asked, in all our years, what my Dad said to him. But I asked him then.

"Nahh, I can't tell you that girl. He said I should keep that between us men." Then solemnly, in a whisper and through his tears, he went on, *"Gi, in so many ways your Dad made me a man. He helped me grow up. I loved him."*

Frankie's funeral was stately. He had a military burial and was laid to rest near his older brother.

I don't know that there's ever a way to prepare for the untimely death of a parent.

I'm not the only one who's lost a parent, or a spouse, or a child or any other dearest loved on in an untimely fashion, and I don't pretend to have the market on sorrow brought by death. I am not a participant in pain Olympics.

But what I do know is that with Frankie's leaving, I welcomed unspeakable grief, terror, uncertainty, and anguish.

Hello Black Night.

BEAUTIFUL

Chapter 5

Having Decided

This we know for sure. Breaking up is hard to do. No doubt. Spend ten years with your high school sweetheart and the ending of your "first love" will indeed be brutal. It's the kind of pain that Phyllis Hyman and Stevie Wonder sang about, the kind of pain that dull aches even decades later. The kind of pain that can only come out by prayer.

Add to that the death of your father, less than a year after the ending of what was an epic love story (in your mind at least) and it would be enough to drive any one to their knees in prayer.

My mother is woman of deep faith.

When she moved to New York City from South Carolina at age 17, one of the very first things she did was to find herself a church and place immediate membership. She made sure that we had a solid, sure Christian education. She made certain that we knew God and His Word. It was her mission to ensure that she would *"train up a child in the way he should go and when he is old, he will not depart from it."* (Proverbs 22:6). It was her focus that we would come to believe in God and understand basic Christian tenants.

My mother is also a pragmatist. She has also made clear that she knew that she was raising two humans who would soon become adult women who could make choices and decisions for themselves. With that, in the healthiest way, she allowed us to "find our own way" in our respective faiths. When we were little girls, she paved the way for us such that there would be no disputing about our foundation, but she was NEVER going to be the one to force God, Christ, the Bible, Christian principles, or Christian living down our throats. That's just not how Sinobia is set up. She is 100% a *"lead the horse to water"* and see what they do with it, kind of Mom. She believed in teaching us "how to fish" in order to help establish our self-sufficiency and she is not one to coddle. Her no-nonsense style of nurturing helped (and really allowed) us to find our way - - bumps, bruises, and REALLY dumb decisions and all.

That said, as a teen, although I had this foundation of faith, I, personally, (through my actions and decisions) was not living for God in the way that the Bible describes. From a Biblical perspective (and I do take the Bible as my standard; my guide) I was far, far, far away from a Christian lifestyle in my relationship with Mr. Young Man. FAR away. And it wasn't like this was unbeknownst to me. What I mean by that is that I knew …FULL WELL…that matched against what I believed the Bible said to be true about relationships (particularly sex before marriage), was NOT how I was living or behaving in my dealings with Mr. Young Man.

Let's pause here. These are my personal beliefs. I am sharing my faith with you – not indicting or judging ANYONE. This was the truth set up for me and what I believed to be the right way to live. For me. #Carryon).

As I was saying, for much of that relationship I lived in a state of guilt at worst – often feeling very far away from God and what I believed to be right.

That said, when things shook out in those very heavy events:

Mr. Young Man and I ka-put…

Frankie having passed away…

Somewhere in me I felt desperate for peace and for answers. I was grieving and brokenhearted and wanted (and needed) direction.

But you know what I cannot stand? I can't stand those kinds of people who only know you when they need you. I ABHOR that behavior. I do my very best to remove myself from folks like that. They strike me as selfish, and self-involved, fully self-absorbed, and self-concerned - - users.

However, if I'm honest, this is precisely how I felt like I had treated God.

Oh, so you know me when you need to get out of bind, huh? You know me when your heart is shattered and torn and you've nowhere else to go, I see.

You'll come and pray to me when your cute tall boy and that earthly Dad (the Dad 'I' gave you by the way) are no more I suppose. NOW you remember me, huh.

These are thoughts that 'I' thought, God thought.

But if we make the choice to believe the Bible, this is not the God that is described *in the Bible*. What God actually says is that when you are at your lowest... when you are your *most* broken... you can come to Him. In fact, two of my favorite scriptures say:

"The Lord is close to the brokenhearted and saves those who are crushed in spirit" (Psalm 34:18) *and "Come close to God and He will come close to you"* (James 4:8).

So, during this black night that's what I did. I cried out to God. I asked Him for help. I asked Him to get me through 'this.' Now, truthfully, there was so much going on with me (so much sadness, so much loss) I didn't actually know what I was asking for help...for, but I still cried out.

Additionally, even with my mother sharing that we needed to know about God, knowing about God... and coming close enough to Him to know Him personally, (intimately), are two different things.

For so long this concept alluded me.

It wasn't until honestly, (and "ironically"), the year before Frankie's death that I really sat down with some friends and studied out some things in the Bible that helped me to see God in a personal and intimate way – not just in the way I learned about Him in church... or in Catholic school.

With these friends, we studied the Word of God to get an understanding about what the Bible says about itself. Next, we went on to study the cross of Christ where, for the first time in my life, I was illuminated about crucifixion and what actually (scientifically) happens to the body if crucified. We learned too why Christ even chose this manner of death and what all that meant. They showed me about the sacrifice of his life and what all that had to do with me having a relationship with God. I went on to learn about how the way that I turned my back on God, the way that I often missed the mark, got in the way of the very relationship that Jesus died to provide for me. I learned a lot about the darkness of this world, and the light of this world, and how to tell the difference. I learned what it means to walk in the light with God, and what that even takes - - and how to recognize what's in the darkness and how to pursue the light. I learned also, and this was so interesting to me, what it meant to *really* follow Jesus. I say that because really following Jesus is actually just the definition of what it means to being a disciple of Jesus. But for me when I heard about the term 'discipleship' initially, I thought - - but isn't "being a disciple' for those guys walking around him in their 'Jesus sandals'?" How can one be a disciple of Jesus in these modern times? I asked these questions only because, at the time, I was confused about what it fully meant to follow Christ. Like, following in his footsteps. figuring out how to be like him. And figuring out why you *would even want to be* like him. I learned with these friends too how we can estimate what it will take to live a life for God and how starting a relationship where we are following Jesus and then stopping in the middle of that journey - - could be unhelpful and harmful.

I was so grateful to my friends for sharing the good news with me and I decided to not only follow Christ – but to be baptized.

No doubt, although I was in great pain, it was beautiful time indeed, so beautiful to hear that there was hope that I could have.

But I messed up. I went about things the wrong way.

Instead of me growing closer to understanding who **_God is and how He could heal me_**, instead, I threw myself into "church." I became a quintessential good single church girl. Bible talks on Tuesday – great! I'll lead it. Mid-week services on Wednesdays – awesome. I'll be there _right_ after work! Helping other people learn about God every other night of the week – SUPER, what time you want me there?

Here's Gigi... reporting for "Christian activity" duty to serve with and on: the singles ministry, the part singers (praise and worship team) ministry, the decorating ministry, the set-up ministry, the break-down ministry, the clean-up ministry, the children's ministry, the babysitting ministry, the "help-this-sister-out-because-she-got-her-heartbroken-like-you-did" ministry, the "help-THIS-sister-out-because-she-lost-her-Daddy-or-her-Mama-suddenly-and-tragically-too" ministry. That's all the ministries ya'll got?!

Any more ministries I can be a part of? Somehow in my psyche I reasoned that I could "busy" my pain away.

Before long I became the busiest girl in the church. Oh, and it fed my ego too – no doubt. *"Oh, Gigi's such a servant..."* or *"Oh, we KNOW Gigi will babysit, she's so reliable, she loves God so much!"* ...or *"Is Gigi free we know she'll help us?"* And, by the way, this "busy-ment" left no room in my life for anything else like reading or writing or creating or... *sleeping.*

I blame no one for this time. It was all me. As a single woman in God's church, I WANTED to serve and WANTED to be a help. This was absolutely true. But I was also hiding. I was telling myself that I was doing all things to be a good Christian (God had asked NONE of this of me...#NONEofIT) but I was using God. I was using the church and the way it was going down, I was helping people out, so who was going to turn me down if I volunteered for 15 simultaneous ministries?

Nan a person. Of course they would take the help!

I think it's dangerous when people are in deep depression or are struggling with grief that is traumatic that we try to push religion, *of any kind*, down their throats. That's not helpful. Its also not helpful to use the machinations of religion, (or the busy doings of ANY organization if we really talking), as a way to mask our pain. That's not helpful either.

What I hope *is* helpful, is helping people to understand that a balm *can* be found in God's arms. But if in fact we choose Christianity, we have to see that the real beauty of God is that we are not required to do all that running around and tiring ourselves out to please Him. Grace, the concept where we receive favor and acceptance from God without having to earn it… unmerited favor if you will, allows us to get to God and not have to do any of that.

For me, while I had indeed decided to follow Christ, I had also decided to ignore my emotional wounds and disastrously misuse church "activities" to help me escape the great pains that laid unresolved in my heart. This only served to hurt me further without leading to *any real healing. It just made everything feel WORSE.*

What I wish I would have focused on during this time – after hearing about the 'beautiful' news of the gospel – was how the Bible and understanding who God is as a Spirit *could have* provided me HOPE.

Again, as I share this, it is not my intention in these pages to push my faith or my religion down anyone's throat, in no way shape or form. But if I'm going to be all the way vulnerable with you, I want to be vulnerable about the only place, in the only way that I've been able to receive relief from my emotional storms. I also want to be open about the fact that although there were indeed instances where I encountered folks who were NOT being kind and Christ-like, my time "in the church" *could have been* a healing place. It could have been a place where I allowed God to soothe and ease my sorrows, but I was hiding out. I wasn't ACTUALLY giving God my heart… but rather using the construct that is "church" (services, many places to serve, fellowship with others) as a numbing agent.

Much like how some use drugs or alcohol.

But none of that was God's fault. I believe that the place for the most healing IS with God. I also have come to believe that grief and loss and heart ache and trauma are allowed to come to us for different reasons. I'd be lying to you if I said I knew what those reasons were. But mayhaps, some of it comes *so that* we can turn to God.

Some pain seems to be inexplicable. WHY DID THIS HAPPEN? Why did this person leave me? Why did this person need to die? Why did I get fired? Why did I get cancer? But faith is inexplicable as well. In fact, the biblical definition of faith *is being sure of what you hope for and certain of what you do not see.*

Very soon after these first really big losses, I DID see that balm and solace and comfort COULD be found in God. However, I had so much "stuff" in my heart and my mind to unpack I dug my heels into the "busy-ment" that can be found in church… rather than digging my heels into the good news. I've shared *"how BEAUTIFUL are the feet of them that preach the Gospel of peace and bring glad tidings of good things!"*

(Romans 10:15)

The "Good News" was to be found in the hope of God and that was BEAUTIFUL.

Running away from my pain was not beautiful.

And that's what I was doing.

Church activity had become my drug of choice.

And not only wasn't that beautiful, but it also wasn't even cute.

Chapter 6

Mi Querida Hermana

(*My Dear Sister*)

I cherish friendship. True and real friendships.

The passage, "*greater love has no one than this: to lay down one's life for one's friends*" (John 15:13), has always meant the greatest deal to me.

Some would say, "Who cares who your friends are? Be a friend to yourself."

Uhmm, okay, sure.

But I have always believed that living in a house by the side of the road WITHOUT being a friend to man made no sense. I have also always believed that, for certain, we need one another.

I've shared with you the friendships that are my life's blessings:

The "J's" – Joyce and Jeanine.

My childhood best friends. Women with whom I have remained friends with to this day. Jeanine and I are in each other's lives DAILY and we have been besties since we were

8 years old.

I treasure that. I honor that.

I also honor the sweet surprise gifts of friendship that I have received later in life.

I have been gifted with a special friend.

Becoming friends with Perla Garcia in our thirties was one such gift.

I met Perla in church.

As part of the same congregation, we had certainly known each other in passing, and had become quite friendly over the years. We ended up at the same single luncheons after service many Sundays

On one such Sunday, while my car was in the shop, I hitched a ride with a married couple in our congregation that lived nearby to get to service but had been offered a ride with the singles to go to lunch with them and other single folks.

It was the custom for a bunch of the singles to find a restaurant after church and sit for hours while eating, laughing, talking, and fellowshipping. On this afternoon, Perla and I ended up sitting next to one another and our laughter was non-stop. The brothers were being particularly entertaining that day and Perla was cracking jokes in my ear. After laughing at one particularly silly comment, I remarked in Spanish,

"*¡Qué cómico!*" (That's funny!)

Shocked, Perla pulled back in her seat and said "*¡Chica, tu hablas español?*" (Girl, do you speak Spanish?!) I replied with my best Bronx "street" Spanish that I had learned while growing up in the Bronx.

Perla was impressed and said she would help me learn more.

From that day, I am not entirely sure how we started hanging out all the time after that, but I do remember that Perla was in my life constantly from that moment on.

We talked on the phone quite a bit during the week, shared Scriptures with each other, rode to church together, and sometimes we met up before our Wednesday night midweek service. It seemed like from soon after that luncheon, we were together all the time.

What we had in common was that we were both young women in the church who were single and over 35 years old at the time. As a matter of fact, over the course of about the next five, six, or even seven years, Perla and I found ourselves in the same Bible discussion group repeatedly for the over 30 to 35 age group.

We would crack up about this all the time. Perla would often say, "there's not a lot of old Broads in the church, Gigi, so its' always going to be me and you."

That wasn't entirely true because there were a few other young ladies in our congregation who were also

180

over 30, close to 35, or even a little older, but Perla was right – there were not many of us.

One of the things that I appreciated about being single and "more mature" was that Perla and I had tons of experiences from before our time in the church that we could share and relate to. Many of those experiences had to do with our families and careers, but others had to do with men and past relationships. We both understood hurt and heartache and spoke openly and vulnerably with each other through the course of our friendship about how God could help us.

Perla did get on me often though about how busy I was all the time, always running around doing this thing or the other. That wasn't her way.

She was very quiet, kept to herself, and although she was definitely a servant, she was a humble and quiet one. Perla had no need to be seen or overly recognized. In large measure, she accepted and loved her station in life. She was very much the definition of being content in every circumstance.

She loved her family so much. On Friday nights, she would often invite me over to spend time with her and her sister as they watched TV or had big dinners with her cousins who came over to just spend time together.

She was generous in her spirit and generous with her life.

Perla also had very little interest in church leadership.

Again, if she was asked to serve or lead, she certainly would, but it wasn't necessary for her to be up in front or have her name called.

At one point, she and I were both in the same Bible discussion group and were asked to co-lead the group together.

That was perfect for us, as we already spent so much time together anyway. She was one of my dearest friends and it made sense. The only thing that posed a problem was that Perla complained she could never find me because I was always off doing something for some other ministry somewhere in the church.

"Aye Gigi… You are so busy. You're busy doing what? … *Mija* (honey, dear, daughter), you need to slow down. What are you hiding from?"

Perla was good at dropping very direct questions to you, no problem.

I would usually ignore her.

I loved that we had different personalities. I was far more extroverted, and you could always find me fellowshipping for hours after service.

Again, that just wasn't Perla's way. She was kind and very giving, but you weren't going to ever find her running around in people's faces. We did love doing the singles lunch after service on Sundays. It was a staple in our church culture, and it felt very stabilizing. It was something we always looked forward to.

Not long after I was asked to lead a Bible discussion with Perla, we were asked to go to lunch with a group of single girls who were also leading Bible discussion groups. This wasn't unusual, necessarily, but we often spent time with the brothers *and* the sisters together. On this particular Sunday, it was just us girls. There were about six of us and we decided that we would all go to a popular local diner to eat and talk before we headed off to a leadership meeting.

As we sat down at the table, there was another young single woman with us who had a reputation for speaking her mind very directly. Sometimes, her comments could be harsh. While we were at the table and while everyone began receiving their lunch order, Perla said, "Everyone: we should congratulate Gigi for being asked to co-lead the discussion with me... *Mija*, I'm so glad to have you in our leadership group. I thank God for you."

The young woman who was known for speaking her mind directly was the first to speak after Perla's comments.

She said, "Yeah, Perla... I'm glad you brought that up. I've been meaning to say something to Gigi about you guys co-leading together. I want to give you a piece of advice Gigi."

Oh Lord. What's this going to be about, I thought.

184

The young lady who liked to speak her mind continued,

"We all know how you are Gigi... always hugging people, always trying to make friends... always being chatty. If you think the way to lead God's people is by using your charm and personality, you're absolutely wrong. You need to know the Bible and show people from the Bible how to follow God. Following God is not all about hugs and personality, so I'm going to tell you right now, if that's the kind of church leader you think you're going to be, you won't do well."

The table fell silent.

This young lady was facing me, sitting directly across from me on the other side of the table. A dear friend was sitting to her immediate left and Perla was sitting at the very end on the other side. I could see 'P' looking at me diagonally across the table, and I could feel that she was willing me not to cry.

I was embarrassed. I didn't understand the harsh admonishment.

I wasn't sure why it was necessary for me to receive this piece of unsolicited advice so publicly at a lunch table. I also wasn't sure how to respond. I wanted to be like Jesus. But I also wanted to lay this chick out.

I was debating.

What if I _DID_ use my personality? Wasn't that what God would have me do? What was her problem? It was obviously my personality.

One of the consequences I found at that time, though, from not dealing with past hurts and having unresolved pain, was that I didn't always deal with my emotions very well in the moment.

I found myself either blowing up at people because I became short and irritated, or just shutting down. Shutting down at this lunch table was now in process.

The young lady that was sitting in between Perla and the sister who spoke her mind finally said, "I think that's enough. I think Gigi has got the point."

What point? Why was her tongue lashing even necessary?

I didn't speak up for myself. I didn't respond at all. There was a part of me that thought that this is what Jesus would have me do - - keep my mouth shut. However, I only internalized the moment, and a venomous anger began to brew.

I had encountered Christian people in the church who were harsh before or whose behavior certainly didn't match the Bible or the fruits of the Spirit, but this seemed to come out of nowhere and was highly inappropriate. It was a painful and embarrassing Moment that taught me the hard way that "church hurt" was real.

All told, at that point in my life, I recognized that I had some: attachment anxiety, relationship grief, grief from death, and also a healthy dose of church hurt.

Terrific.

After lunch, we all went to our cars. Perla started walking quickly to catch up to me as she could see that

I was separating myself from the group. As I got to my car door, she put her hand on my shoulder and said,

"Look, ignore her, okay? Why didn't you say anything?"

"Say anything, like what, Perla? I didn't want to look like I was being defensive, and I certainly didn't understand where all that was coming from."

My dear friend Perla then imparted on me a piece of wise and sage advice that I've never forgotten:

"Gigita, I watch you sometimes and I wonder why on earth you feel like you have to be everywhere. Sometimes, I watch you and wonder if something is inside of you that makes you feel like you must please everyone. I don't know, Mama, so I'm not accusing you of this, but sometimes I wonder if you say yes to everything because you want or need people to like you. I think that you have lost so many people in your life that you don't want to lose other people, so you do things, and you say yes because you think that's going to make people like you more.

I don't know, but sometimes that's what I think. I think something happened to you when you were in the Bronx before you came here to New Jersey, that you never talk about. Sometimes I think that comes out in the way that you are in the church. But Mijita, God loves you just for you and ONLY for you. I know this, for sure. You don't have to do anything or prove anything to anyone, and you don't have to be afraid of Him leaving you. He won't and I won't either. I don't know why this girl felt the need to say those things but ignore them. God made you who you are for a reason, and he loves you for that."

Perla was onto something, that's for sure.

But I wasn't ready to cop to any that.

I gave her a big hug and thanked her for her wisdom and love.

I had to work through some serious steps to forgive the girl with the direct tongue.

Not long after that, Perla and I were asked to be bridesmaids in the wedding of a beloved sister in the church. We had been given the details for the dress that we should go and get from David's Bridal to get fitted before the wedding. We had an appointment two weeks prior, but Perla had been under the weather, and we ended up not going. On this particular Saturday, we met for lunch and headed over to David's Bridal for the fitting. While she was in the dressing room, she asked me to come and zip up the back of her dress. When I did, I could see that she had lost an inordinate amount of weight. This wasn't the first time I had noticed it, but when zipping up the back of her dress, I was shocked to see how thin she was.

"P, what's the matter with you?"

"Aye Gigi, por favor... I'm fine"

But Perla was certainly not fine.

She was actually very ill. She was so ill, in fact, that the very next day she was admitted to the hospital. Two days went by, then three, then a week, and Perla was still in the hospital.

Before long, it became very clear to me that her illness was far more serious than she had let on. During this time, her sister asked if I would be willing to be a part of their family rotation and stay over with Perla at the hospital one night of the week.

Each of Perla's sisters, and some of her cousins, would each take a night to ensure that Perla wasn't alone through the night. There was one Friday night, where the family needed coverage to make sure that Perla had company. Her sister said to me, "Gigi, you know how my sister is. She's so private and there are only a couple of people she would want to stay with her. Do you think you can keep her company on Friday nights?"

Her family didn't even have to ask.

Almost immediately, along with Perla's sisters, I became a part of her family rotation and spent time with her in the hospital each Friday night.

It was kind of cool because we usually did our single girls thing on Friday nights anyways. But these visits were very special. They often consisted of me reading her Psalms from the Bible or us singing hymns together. She loved the song, "Humble Yourself in the Sight of the Lord and He Will Lift You Up."

We sung that often.

Four more weeks went by, and Perla was still in the hospital. It became known to us that she was probably not going to make it out. During the week her health most significantly declined, I received an urgent call at work from her sister encouraging me to get to the hospital that night.

It wasn't a Friday night, it was a Thursday night, so it wouldn't have been a night that I would be ordinarily come visiting. This was a different night. It was a gathering and a time for farewells of sorts.

When I arrived, a social worker (someone I had seen many evenings during my visit with Perla), said in the hallway, "It might be a good idea to start saying your goodbyes. We don't suspect that she'll have many more days. We do think she's holding on, though, so if you're close to her, you should convince her to let go."

My God.

When I went into the room, all of Perla's cousins and some of her coworkers and girls from church were in the room, as well. Our ministry leader was there reading scriptures. While you could hear people softly crying, it was the strangest thing because even though we knew that Perla's illness was winning out, on this particular night, she had a bit more alertness through her.

She was such a feisty one. She sat up and said, "What is everyone doing here?!"

We all cracked up.

Perla was bossing us around, as usual.

After talking with her sisters and cousins, one of her sisters said, "P, Gigi is here... you see her?"

Her eyesight had begun to dim.

She called me over to her and said... "My *Gigita*, remember what I taught you, okay, *Hermana*? You don't need to prove anything to anyone. God loves you just for you. Only for you. You don't need to be running around. Something is hurting you. Stop running from it, okay? Mama, you must stop. And Gigi, the things that are hurting you inside you have to talk it out, okay? Okay?"

As you might imagine, I could barely respond.

Even as I recount this, I can barely breathe now. How was this happening? How was my dear sister, such a pure soul, leaving this world?

But for certain, for absolute certain, Perla was ready. She loved God so much and she had recently told me on a Friday night together in the hospital that she had no regrets. She had nothing left on her heart and she was ready to be with God.

How was it that she was thanking me when it was *me* that should've been thanking her?

She recognized in me that all was not well. Perla was not afraid to say so. That wasn't the first time that she had suggested to me that I get help for whatever was going on with me. It wasn't the first time that we had talked about people pleasing, stuffing down feelings, or other things that she could detect in me. She knew something was deeply troubling me and there was something about getting this admonishment from my dear sister on her way home to the Lord that stuck with me.

Perla recognized that I had a lot of grief and sadness from loss in my heart. Now compounded, I would have to deal with the loss of my friend, as well.

On the next night, Perla gave up her spirit and quietly passed away. Her parents and her faithful sisters were in the room. I was there, too. In the Moment that she left, the room was nearly silent, but it was quite obvious that her spirit had gone to take her rest. It was soul crushing and quite beautiful all at the same time.

There are many beautiful things that have defined my relationship with God and my friendship with Perla, because of who she was and how she loved, is one. of those things.

What's more, I thank God for her life-saving message to me:

"Take care of yourself, Mama. Talk it out and go get help. God loves you so much."

And my message to her?

"Gracias por todo mi querida hermana, y gracias por tu vida. Yo siempre te amare y ni por un segundo te descuidare," (Thank you for everything my dear sister, and thank you for your life. I'll always love you and not for a moment can I forget you).

GET WELL

Chapter 7

Helpless and Harassed

L uckily, I could still get into my old apartment. Three weeks before Perla 's passing, I moved to a new place.

It was somewhat of an old place turned new place.

I had been living with Keischa before she and Orlando got married. Keischa was one of the best roommates I ever had. We decided to move in together for several reasons. The largest benefit was Keischa's amazing knowledge and focus on health as a training professional. I became my most healthy self when living with Keischa. I was my most healthy self, *physically*, that is.

I was going to the gym regularly, eating with discipline and intention, and had lost a great deal of weight. Keischa was tremendously supportive of that.

We had a wonderful household full of love, laughter, honesty, and safety. She and Orlando ((her boyfriend and now, longtime husband) were absolutely family to me.

As such, naturally, when it became obvious that they needed to move up their wedding date, and Keischa asked if I would be willing to break our lease early, I was happy to oblige.

She had also asked me, along with her older biological sister, to stand up for her at her wedding. I was thrilled to be her maid of honor and I was happy to help her and Orlando in any way that I could.

In the immediate term, which meant moving out of our lovely two-bedroom condo so they could move forward properly with their wedding plans.

As God would have it, a unit in my old complex became available. I'd be moving into a new unit, but back to the same condo complex where I had once lived. It tickled me that the complex was called "Queens Square." And be sure that I absolutely took that as a wink from God.

So, during Perla's last days, I was also moving.

My last piece of furniture to move (my extra-long couch), required movers who were not available on the afternoon the afternoon I needed them. With that, I arranged with our old property owner to leave my big couch in the old apartment for another couple of weeks and move it out before the end of the month. Aside from the couch, the apartment was emptied out.

The night that Perla passed away, even though Keischa had already moved out, and the place was hollow, I opted to stay there and sleep on the couch. Either way, in my new spot or back at the old one, I was going to be alone. I guess I just didn't want to be alone in the new spot. There was something still so comforting and warm about the place I shared with Keischa.

I grabbed an overnight bag and back went to our old place. I had the keys until month's end, and it almost felt like a place to hide.

It just so happens, that I had arranged the next day for the movers to come and get the couch to move to my new place, anyway, so this last night in our old place seemed to make sense.

Except, I soon realized that an empty apartment when you are grieving only makes matters worse. It seemed like I cried incessantly that night before tiring myself out on the couch.

I struggled to get myself going the next morning and I could almost feel the depression setting in. I tried to push through it.

I had a ton of phone calls to make and a few errands to run that Perla's sister had asked me to help them out with. I had a lot to do, actually – what else was new?

I was indeed listless and had very little sleep the night before because of the sobbing, tossing and turning, and reliving every Moment of the evening before. With the passing Moments, I felt myself sinking deeper into a pit of sadness.

That's the thing about grief and loss. One big loss calls up all the haunts and forgotten emotions of every other loss before it.

And then, don't mess around and not properly face or deal with any of those *first* losses. By the time, your heart is in pain again, that pain is intensified, combined, and packed together like an explosive.

Finally, I got up and took a shower and put my things back in my overnight bag and got dressed. I was just in time because the movers were just arriving to come get the couch.

I was grateful for the brief distraction and knew I had to go home and unpack my new place and get my life together.

But that's not what happened.

When I got to my new place (in the old complex), I finished up making those phone calls and I laid RIGHT back down on the couch. I was lethargic and had little to no appetite. I was tearful with no desire to connect, talk, or socialize. All I wanted was the comfort of my big squishy couch.

I did not move for the next couple of days.

I had boxes to unpack and phone calls to return, but I did none of that. I turned the TV on, eventually, but for the most part, I just laid on the couch, lights off, curtains drawn sleeping, sitting, crying, trying to read my Bible, giving up, and laying back down again.

There was no peace.

The dark spirits of despondency were on me like a shroud, and they were not letting up. It reminded of the passage of scripture in Matthew 9:36, *"When he saw the crowds, he had compassion on them, because they were harassed and helpless, like sheep without a shepherd."*

I felt helpless…and certainly felt very harassed.

When Sunday came, I needed to decide whether to go to church. I was dreading it. I knew that there would be lots of talk of Perla and the services and requests to pray for her family. These were the only things I was managing to do, but I certainly was not in the mood for any questions. People knew that she was one of my dearest friends and that I had spent a lot of time with her and her family in the hospital. I anticipated the well-meaning, albeit awkward, comments, questions, and expressions of sympathy. I believe that those expressions of sympathy were ill-placed because I was more concerned about Perla's family than anything.

Early Sunday morning the phone rang.

It was my mother.

"How come I didn't hear from you the last few days Miss-Missy? I know you're sad, but you can't hide away. Are you going to church?"

I sighed slowly. My mother had Gigi radar.

I'm quite sure that I was in the same clothes I had been in for the previous few days as I remember being aware of myself.

"Well... I'm not sure about going to church yet, but I certainly need a shower."

I mentioned to you earlier that my mother is a pragmatist. Her heart is filled with love for her kids, but her process in getting us going, has always been – TO GET US GOING. Aside from that, there is never a scenario in my mother's world where _not_ attending service would have been an option.

"Yeah, you better take a shower. And while you're at it, put some coffee on, pull out your outfit, and make the decision that you are GOING TO GET UP AND GO PRAISE GOD. From what you told me; your friend Perla was a woman of faith. She is safe now and all will be well for her. If you don't take care of *yourself*, you'll be next and I'm in no mood to bury you. You need to hear from God, so get to service."

Nothing like a no-nonsense kind of Mom, boy.

I took my mother's advice, dragged myself into the kitchen, and figured out which of the un-opened boxes had my coffee maker. I pulled it out, put on a pot of coffee, went to shower, and got dressed. Our service was about 20 minutes away from the new condo. In Central Jersey though, we used to say that everything was 20 minutes away from *everything*, so I didn't have far to go.

I put on a pair of black slacks and my favorite gray and black sweater. I wasn't intending to dress like I was in mourning. Those were just the pieces that I had available on hand.

I had already washed my face and put on a dusting of foundation powder with the slightest bit of lip gloss, but I needed to make my hair look like something.

I went back to the bedroom to get some hair product. When I returned to the bathroom and ran the comb through my hair, for the second time in my adult life, I looked down in the bathroom sink and staring back up at me was more than two fistfuls of my own hair.

A couple of years earlier, I had been diagnosed with Sarcoidosis which had many symptoms. I was never quite sure if, or when, hair loss might be a part of that, but I certainly knew from previous bouts (of what felt like depression), that hair loss was not uncommon for me when I was in this state. Hair loss had also been a hereditary thing from Dad's side of the family... so between the sarcoid and my family traits my poor little follicles couldn't catch a break.

In this instance, though, there was an inordinate amount of hair in my comb and in the sink. The sight was horrifying, as you might imagine.

As I gripped the sides of the vanity, I felt utter panic well up in me as I could see the wide spaces in my scalp. This time, the tears came easily again, and I heard myself whimper out to God.

"Father, please... please help me. I'm in bad shape. I'm in really bad shape. I'm not going to make it Lord. Please. My hair is falling out again..."

I was weeping again.

I managed to use enough hair product to slick back what was left of the hair on top of my head into the semblance of a bun. But if you looked right at me, you could see where the hair had fallen out in big patches. I wasn't going to get away with this style, so I threw on a cap and left.

I was starting to run late.

When I got to the service, as I suspected, I ran into folks in the parking lot right away. "Oh Gigi, how are you? How's Perla's family doing? Do you know when the services are going to be?" All reasonable questions and these good Christians were well-meaning and showing great compassion. "Let's just keep praying for them as they've been through a lot. I think we'll get more information about the services in the next couple of days." I was careful not to answer anything about myself. I wasn't trying to go there, and I was not in the mood to be open.

I got inside the building and there was more of the same. Warm, sympathetic, and loving Christians all very sad at the passing of our dear sister.

Be outward, Gigi, I told myself.

Focus on others.

This is not about you.

You still need to be giving to Perla's family. Remember that.

As I moved into the sanctuary and looked to take my seat, one of the single girls who had recently gotten engaged bounded up to me with great enthusiastic energy.

"Hey girl!! I wanted to make sure that you had gotten this." Even before she put it in my hand, I believe that I suspected what it was. Without thinking, I snarled at her in response.

"What is this?" But I already knew.

People were unaccustomed to getting any tone from me except for a warm, cheerful, and often gregarious greeting. And I was known in the church for my love for weddings. I had been a bridesmaid at that point 17 times. All told, since then, I've been a bridesmaid 20 times. My name was synonymous with weddings so if newly engaged bride to be in the church expected anyone to be happy for her – it would have been me.

I know that my snarl was jarring and hurtful to her.

She was so startled that she hesitated in her reply.

"Well… well… it's… it's…" Oh man, she was startled all right, stuttering, and taken aback by my tone.

"It's our wedding invitation?" Which she said in a questioning tone.

"I can see that." I shot back.

Hurt people, hurt people. I was acting terribly.

This young lady was immediately perceptive. "Gigi, have I offended you?" Underneath all the sadness and despair and I don't even know what else I was feeling, I was angry. I was angry at God, Frankie, Mr. Young Man, the girl at the lunch table, and I was angry at every other *anything* that had ever slighted me, injured me, or left me sad. Or had - - just left me; like had abandoned me. I was mad, that's for sure, and unfortunately, this young new bride-to-be was about to get the brunt of it.

"You do know that Perla is dead, don't you?"

Oy. I was brutal.

The young sister was aghast. It was in her face, but I could see her hand shaking as she didn't know what to do with her wedding invitation – or what to say to me.

She apologized profusely and somewhere during her apology the Holy Spirit got a hold of me and my conscience was pricked: I felt lower than an inchworm. I told her, "No, I'm sorry. You're planning for your wedding, and you have every right to be excited and every right to hand out your wedding invitations today at church. I'm just in such a bad way."

She said she understood and asked if I wanted to take the invitation or not. I felt like vermin. I had ruined this girl's Moment of happiness. I did attend her wedding in the coming weeks and she and I became really good friends following that exchange, but not until after having a chat about how horrible I was to her in that Moment. She was gracious to forgive me, thank God, but I would find myself responding and reacting to many people like this over the course of the next several weeks.

Some weeks after Perla's home-going service, I was asked to serve at a few events. It just so happened that all three of these events were taking place on the same day. It never even crossed my mind to say no. I was thrilled for the distraction. This was my M.O. (and the very thing that Perla cautioned me against, by the way) to hide from what I was really feeling.

I had been asked that morning to go to the church fellowship hall and set up for a repast. I did so and although it hadn't been asked of me, I stayed around to help clean up. From there, I was asked to go and decorate for a baby shower that was happening for a pregnant sister in the congregation. I packed up my car after the early morning repast and headed over to where the baby shower was happening to set-up the decorations and make sure that everything looked 'just so.'

From there, there was an event happening at our ministry leader's house that evening. He and his wife had asked me to come by their house and help them set up. I arrived at their house before they did and sat in my car as I waited for them to get home.

As they drove up to the house, the ministry leader said, "How on earth did you beat us here? We were all just at the same event, Gigi!

And how is it that you have unloaded all the decorations from the baby shower and yet your car is *re-loaded* with all of the things for tonight?"

I chuckled, shrugged, and joked, "Come on, man, you know my car is a clown car. You know, the kind used in the circus where there are 5, 10, maybe 15 clowns that fit in to one car and you can't figure out how so many are still pouring out. That's what this is. Hahaha."

We shared a belly laugh over it.

Like usual, I played it off. This was the response I typically gave to people when they asked me how I fit so many things in my car and how I was able to zip from one event to the other undetected and laser focused on my contrived busy church work. I went in with them and helped set up for the evening's event. Folks started to arrive, we fellowshipped, and enjoyed the evening together. Afterwards, I stayed to help clean up. I had been on the go from 6 AM and I was finishing up now at nearly midnight.

I was exhausted, but at least I didn't have to think. I certainly didn't have to *feel*.

The following day was Sunday. I got to church and wanted to go in for the message, but I was really not in the mood to fellowship.

When service was over, I packed my things quickly and I made a B-line for the door. Just as I was moving up the aisle towards the back door, I heard our ministry leader call out asking if he could chat with me for a few.

This was curious to me. He was the head Pastor. He had a whole church to think about. Although we were really good friends, and he and his wife were two people I very much trusted (and very much loved), I couldn't understand why he was taking time out of his busy fellowship schedule to talk to me.

"Sis. My wife and I went to bed last night very concerned about you. Even though we had that funny 'ha-ha' about your clown car and you arriving to our house before we did after a full day of church events, last night before we went to bed, we were praying, and God put you squarely on our hearts.

Sis, it suddenly dawned on me as I started to think about you and how you move. It occurred to me that you are busier than me and I'm the leader of the church!

I started thinking about you and the last few years and how you move about and how you are everywhere, *all the time*."

In these days, my temper was short, and I could feel a storm of offense brewing right under my skin. The truth is the brother was trying to help me. He and his wife were being thoroughly loving, but I got mad at him.

"You're kidding me, right? You've got to be joking me right now. I'm one of the biggest servants you have in this joint, Bro. There's nothing that you, or your wife, or any of the other church leaders have asked me to do that I don't do. I make myself available. I babysit. I decorate. I set up for weddings, funerals, baby showers, and singles events. I sing with the part-singers (the praise and worship folks) when needed, help in the children's ministry, sit with the old people, sit with the young people and you're not grateful? I'm the hardest working single chick you got up in here, Sir."

When I remember this, in my mind's eye I see our ministry leader looking at me with a face full of compassion. When I thought about the night before when he and his wife were praying about me, they were figuring me out. He started piecing it together and I could see in this Moment that he understood what was really happening.

"Gi, we think you're in trouble. I don't know from what and I don't know how deep it goes, but as your brother in Christ, as your Pastor, and as your friend, Sis, I have to tell you that you're in trouble. Have you ever thought about seeking professional help?"

Oh. This conversation is over.

"Professional help for what? I'm fine."

In my mind, I was thinking, girl, you just spent days alone in your apartment with the curtains drawn, un-showered, a sink full of your own hair, crying, and full of despair. You mean to tell me you can't see that what this brother is saying to you is right? Certainly, you are being harassed by these demonic emotions. Certainly, you are being harassed by the pains of your past. Perla saw it and now you're snapping at people left and right. God has now sent the WHOLE Pastor of the

WHOLE church to leave his flock of fellowship after service, and B-line for you to help you see that you need help, - - but you mad. Ok Gigi.

I promise I had this entire conversation in my head while the Pastor was finishing up his comments. I thanked him for his concern, and I acquiesced to some extent, but only to make it *look* like I was being humble. "Maybe you're right. Maybe I do need help. Maybe I DO have some things that I've never talked about or never healed from. I'm going to pray about it."

My Pastor was extremely generous with me because he knew me well. He smirked a bit because he knew full well that I didn't believe a word of what I had just shared. "Okay, Gigi, let me know if you need help talking things through. My wife and I love you very much and I want to see you get the help you need." My Pastor thinks I'm a lunatic, I thought. Fun times.

Because where Sir, pray tell, was I supposed to get this help?

Chapter 8

Where Do Broken Hearts Go?

T he most logical place to start, I thought, as I contemplated where to go for counseling and therapy assistance, was with my work benefits.

Okay, so let's just say for the sake of argument that I *did* agree to speak to a professional. I wasn't convinced and I certainly wasn't on board, but I had to admit that I felt a little like I was falling to pieces. The hair loss in the sink was the last straw. I was still crying, quite short tempered, and had no desire to talk to anyone about how I was feeling. I was not feeling well, at all.

Someone suggested that I call the Employee Assistance Program (EAP) line offered by my job at that time.

If I'm honest, I don't think that I made a conscious decision that I was going to go in and make a call to our

EAP services, but I could hear the small voice in the back of my head nagging me that I *should* do it. I got to work that Monday and I began my day as normal, but I kept hearing the small voice telling me to call those people.

This went on all day, but I never made the call. Honestly, a week went by and although I thought about it every day, I *still* didn't call. Finally, I gathered the courage to call our benefits administrator.

While on the one hand, the thought of me asking anyone at work about our mental health benefits felt like a bad idea, but I seriously did need a bit more direction on how the EAP worked.

I was at the very early stages of my learning and professional days and as a training specialist, I was folded into the human resources team. That meant that the benefits administrator and I were actually teammates, of sorts. I think this had something to do with my reluctance, but I didn't know where else to turn for the next right next step. I sent her an email, and a couple of hours later she gave me a call. I thought about lying and saying that I was asking for the information for somebody else, but the more I thought it, lying was stupid so I just told the truth.

I kept it easy breezy, though, "Hey Bell, how are you?"

I kept my voice friendly and sweet, certainly not letting on that I had a dark cloud of doom over my head. I asked some vetting questions about the EAP and how to access their services. I asked also if there was a claim process involved and would the claim be anonymous and what it would all entail.

She explained the situation and how I could get into the system.

It would take a few more days, yet but I *finally* made the call.

Essentially, the way the employee assistance program was set up, the first step was to call the EAP 'general' line and explain your situation. If you were someone in need of immediate help you were referred to a hotline or mental health professional with critical urgency. For less acute emotional needs, they connected you with a mental health professional who acted as a guide. This person was more like a concierge if you will. You weren't signing up to have this person as your therapist, but this individual was usually a licensed social worker or psychologist in the early part of their career who would help *to lead you* on the path to finding a therapist.

They also helped to do an assessment to ascertain what might be troubling you.

When I got connected with my first EAP guide, we spent our first few conversations talking through why I believed that I needed this help.

Let's call this guide "Joey."

Joey was a young white man barely 30-years =-old (which put him several years younger than me at the time).

It was clear to me that he was very early in his career.

Great, I thought.

The first time I call EAP services, and I get - - Doogie Houser. #Swell.

Is this my life?

But I was so wrong about those initial thoughts. Joey was great! Really great. His age played no bearing. He was wise, mature, easy to talk to and deeply compassionate. For someone early in his career, he did ask a lot of the right questions. He allowed me to go at my own pace and if at any time I felt unsafe or as if he were pushing, he would pull back.

Our goal together was not to necessarily come up with a treatment plan. Our goal together was for Joey to walk me through an assessment plan or an assessment process where he diagnosed me in a triage kind of way. We worked together to figure out what might be going on with me and then, we found the most appropriate mental health professional in my benefits plan that could potentially help to treat me long-term.

The problem with that was that one of the things that Joey helped to diagnose (and this wasn't surprising to me), was his suspicion that I had an "anxious attachment style." This attachment style means several things about the way I quickly attach to people and how that creates anxiety in me, along with a host of other maladies.

And so wouldn't you know, and here I was, getting attached to Joey!

Doogie Hauser ended up being *exactly* the only person I wanted to talk to. But it didn't work that way. One of the things that I found out throughout this process, in terms of getting help and figuring out where I could get that help, was that I was going to have to keep an open mind and be committed _to the process._

I was overwhelmed and uninterested in either of those options.

I just wanted to talk with Joey.

But alas.

As it happened, Joey did indeed find me three appropriate counselors right off the bat. Besides my anxious attachment style, Joey surmised that I was suffering from at least a form of clinical depression and grief syndrome.

Fair.

The first three counselors that Joey connected me with all specialized in one or two or all three of these unique treatment areas.

We found that that the first psychologist wasn't taking any new patients.

Cool.

The next Provider that he connected me to, was a lady psychologist. She was more mature, and she was a part of the Rutgers community, to some extent. As a Rutgers alum, this set me on a great path to get started. Even though she didn't see patients on the campus of Rutgers, she had an office that was considered to be an extended Rutgers administration facility.

Sweet.

This was great because Rutgers is beloved my alma mater and there was a sense of comfort there. I didn't book right away. I was still struggling with the whole thing. It wasn't so much that I felt stigmatized about getting the help. I think that the real problem was that I felt a sense of embarrassment, deep embarrassment, about needing *to get the help in the first place.*

Words like "crazy," "emotional disorders," "unstable," "cuckoo bird," "loon," and "nut job" were a few labels that I was afraid of and were swirling around in my brain.

But Joey had me all in it now, and if nothing else, I was curious to see how far we could get.

So, I went ahead and made an appointment to finally meet with the lady that was connected to Rutgers University. She and I went back and forth at first trying to find an appropriate meeting time. This was well before we were doing things on Zoom, so this meant a face-to-face appointment in her office.

When I arrived, the outer foyer of the office was everything that my mind expected it to be. Slightly sterile, but serene, and some pieces of furniture that looked like they were *trying* to make you feel more relaxed. For example, on a couch that looked long enough to seat five or six people in the waiting room, there were these big pillows that said "BREATHE," "You're okay," and "One Day At A time."

Hard eyeroll.

I traveled down a dark ominous hallway to her office. I hated the dank and dark hallway, but as I got to her room, there was a huge window wall that let in the sun with incredible brilliance. That was a great sign. I love the light. Having so much natural light come into her office was fantastic.

She had the office set up in a weird way, though. Instead of a seating arrangement where she and I could be face-to-face, her desk sat perpendicular in front of the large picture window, so the window was on her right and her desk was facing the back wall of her office. There was a chair to the right of the desk where the patient could sit, but it was much more like a student coming in to see a professor for office hours.

I could feel that I was hyper-critical, so I told myself not to be so picky.

This was my very first experience with a therapist. Calm down Gi…

What do you know?

I sat down with Eliza, and we began to chat.

She was nice and awfully polite, but I noticed immediately that she was very, very, *very* nervous. As we tried to get to know each other some, I noticed that her hands were shaking, and she was looking all around the office (as if she were looking for someone). She looked around so much, that it caused me to do the same thing (which was highly irrational because it was only her and I in there).

Who was she looking for? What was she experiencing? Her behavior was quite distracting. At one point, as I tried to answer her questions, I saw her look off into the distance and smile wide as if she was smiling at someone on the other side of the room. I reasoned with myself.

Gigi… Don't you dare turn around.

You don't know *who* this lady is smiling at, but you know ain't NOBODY else is here.

Finally, I asked, "Eliza, are you okay?"

What happened next, I was ready for.

Eliza broke down in tears, sobbing and told me a very harrowing tale about a traumatic experience that had just happened to her. The experience had left her anxious and feeling like she was unable to cope.

Everything in me was sparked to compassion.

But truthfully, I thought to myself, is this happening right now? I began to give Eliza some advice. I listened to her story, affirmed her, asked if she had any techniques to calm herself down – and then shared one of my own. Finally, I asked (and not in a way to be snarky or to clown her, but I genuinely concerned),

"Eliza, do you have anyone that *you* can talk to?"

The experience with Eliza taught me one thing.

It taught me to be cognizant of the fact that even the helpers need to be helped. It helped me to see that even the servants need someone to serve them. My heart went out to her because she was clearly struggling. On the other hand, this was certainly not helping my fledgling quest to pursue professional help.

It was what it was.

The next day, I spoke to my boy, Joey, and recounted the visit.

I tried really hard not to laugh until Joey burst out laughing. "Keeping it real," he said, "you know I shouldn't laugh…and I'm not laughing _at_ this lady, Gigi and her situation. But the irony is that we have finally convinced you to go and see someone and YOU do the counseling! That experience was the stuff of a sitcom."

Or maybe a good book. (*wink*)

Joey and I talked again over the next couple of days, and we determined that I would go to the next option on our list.

Hanging in there, I began the process all over again.

I reached out to the professional and set up a meeting time. This provider was a much older white man, and it was clear that he had extensive experience in counseling and treating patients. I was surprisingly not concerned about race or gender. I only say that because there was a point where I thought that I would feel more comfortable with a black woman therapist. This time, it didn't faze me one way or the other. I *was* concerned, however, if this gentleman had experience with single people. I felt like processing my relationship trauma was key to my healing. After asking him a series of questions, I felt satisfied and planned to go see him.

His offices were swanky. I loved that. There was a lovely waiting area outside his office suite, tons of good magazines, and even a few good book titles. There was soft music playing in the foyer, but it wasn't cheesy elevator music. The music was more like smooth jazz with some songs in rotation that had an upbeat tempo every couple of songs.

"Nice touch with the music," I thought.

I got into the expensive looking office, and I immediately noticed his wealth. There were fancy rugs, a beautiful leather couch, beautiful pillows, a gorgeous mahogany desk, beautiful expensive-looking paintings, and lots of lush green plants. Elliott came from behind his desk and ushered me to a "sitting area" he had set up for us to talk. He offered me a seat on the couch and right across from me, he had set up a recliner chair, where he sat. It had a deep back and a high headrest.

Comfy.

As Elliott and I began the conversation, it had some of the same elements as the conversation I had with Eliza. He asked me a lot about my parents, my childhood, my siblings, my birth order, and some other context and background questions.

He asked, "Tell me what brought you here today."

Now, ya'll know I can talk.

If I feel comfortable, I will start my story at the beginning of creation to take you through the end of the world. Truthfully, I wasn't thinking that I should make my stories to the therapist concise because I *wanted* him to know exactly who I was.

However, to my chagrin, after I had been speaking for a bit, I realized that Elliott's eyes were closed. Shut. I mean, I never saw him blinking or trying to hold his eye lids open. You know, like when you're out with a friend and maybe it's late and you can tell that your friend is sleepy and trying to stay awake?

In one Moment, Elliot and I were talking, and in the next... my man was snoring!

He was FAST asleep!

Bwhahahaha!

It would have been hilarious had it not been so unfortunate.

You can't be serious, God. I thought. You can't be. Lord.

But I felt sorry for him. The poor baby was tired.

And I was in there utterly talking to myself.

Not wanting to wake the baby, I wrote a check and left it on the coffee table in his sitting area and let myself out.

For crying out loud. The therapist fell asleep on me.

This wasn't working out for me. This was not working out for me, *at all.*

I called Joey, and this time I had no grins and giggles.

I was irritated. I was agitated. And I was ready to give up.

Judge me if you want because I know I had *only* seen two professionals.

But when you are desperately trying to call up the courage to do a thing you really don't want to do in the first place, two strikes back-to-back were enough to discourage me.

Joey did his best to keep me focused and he asked me to try one more time.

I returned home that afternoon after my encounter with the "sleeping therapist" and I was all parts dismayed and annoyed. I was already talking myself out of the whole thing.

When your ministry leader (your Pastor), gives you a piece of advice, it certainly feels like you *shouldn't* ignore it.

Our ministry leader was my Pastor, and my friend. At that time, he knew me quite well and I had spent a great deal of time with him and his wife, and their kids. There was no doubt in my mind that they cared for me as my family in the faith. I had no reason to believe that he would steer me astray.

But this here WHACK search? This nonsense?!?

This was for the birds.

Yeah, I wasn't with this.

The lady therapist needed *me* to counsel *her*.

She was clearly hurting and struggling on her own. How was she helping me? How was she helping _ANYBODY_? I'm not going to even get STARTED on "Dr. Sleepy."

The thought of Elliott fast asleep cracks me up every time I think about it! But for someone just tenuously deciding that therapy was right for them, his nap time did not spur me on to greatness.

Then, there was the way that I felt about Joey.

I was quite surprised at how well he did his job. His credentials read that he was a LCSW (a licensed clinical social worker) and for a young counselor, he was impressive. I joked at first about his youth, but his wisdom and tenderness were what I believed I needed at that time. He made me feel seen and safe. However, I could not stick with him because that was against the EAP rules.

I was feeling quite frustrated.

As it was, I was not 100% convinced that I believed my ministry leader in the first place. Maybe I was actually just going through a rough patch and really didn't *need* to get help. "Listen to your Pastor" and "you must do this" were messages not resonating with me. Furthermore, it had always been taught to me that, as a

Christian, if you wanted to move through your troubles, you put into practice the acronym of P.U.S.H.

Pray-Until-Something-Happens.

"P.U.S.H." is what I think many Christians had been taught to do. There seemed (and still seams) to be this expectation of the believer that if you believed in God and believed in the Bible that would be all you needed. While I was still personally struggling to see if therapy was right for *ME*, this PUSH business didn't seem like the right thinking to me, either.

Many say that if you love God and you rely on your faith, you will not need to go to therapy.

You won't need to talk to a psychologist…

You won't need to focus on your mental health…

On that, I vehemently and completely disagreed.

Would we tell someone who was diagnosed with congestive heart failure, "Oh, Shuga, just read your Bible…you don't need to see a cardiologist!"

Would we tell someone who was diagnosed with stage IV cancer, "Oh no, honey, just grab yourself a Psalm, hold on to God's unchanging hand, and you'll be fine. You don't need to go to an oncologist!"

No. Of course not. We absolutely would not say these things.

I believe in the process of getting help for mental health issues and concerns, I just wasn't convinced that *I* needed that help.

God provided us with intellect and the ability to reason. Medical professionals, like cardiologists, oncologists, and endocrinologists, have been placed here and have been given their skills to help all of us. In the same way, I believe that God has provided mental and emotional wellness professionals. They are experts that can help us understand, identify, and become aware of patterns and cycles that keep us emotionally unwell and mentally bound.

I believe that helps comes from God.

I believe that HE set all of that up.

I just wasn't sure He set all that up *for me.* Apparently, not.

Eliza needed *me* to counsel *her*... Good God.

And Elliott, "Dr. Sleepy," fell asleep. Mercy.

The one person that I felt was credentialed and caring enough to get in there with me, (although he *did* remind me of Doogie Houser), couldn't connect with me long-term because he couldn't become my therapist of record.

I thought, *you know what?*

I'm good.

After I got home from my visit with Dr. Sleepy, I sat on the couch, and pondered these things. I sat there and felt sorry for myself for a couple of hours. I finally forced myself up from the sofa, pulled off my clothes, and got in my sweats. I could feel myself getting ready for another three days of couch abyss.

Just as I put on my favorite Rutgers t-shirt, my mother called.

Her daughter antennas were on high frequency, goodness.

"What's going on with you, Miss Missy?"

Parents have keen Spidey senses.

My mother's intuition about me has NEVER, EVER been wrong and is always precisely timed. She has also never been one to allow me to give in to my darkest emotions. She is a true parent-coach, and she wasn't about that coddle-my-kid-life.

Ever.

However, I wasn't quite ready to share with her (not in the least, actually), that I had begun a quest for a therapist. I wasn't even ready to tell her that I was considering therapy at all. Like I told you, I wasn't sure about the whole process myself yet.

I gave her a generic answer in response and said, "all good Mom... What's going on with you?"

There was a knowing, very pregnant pause of silence for a Moment, but she said nothing and went on.

Mom always let us come around to share with her when we are ready.

She said,

"You'll never guess who I saw today!"

Oh Lord. Who could she run into?

"I ran into your old bestie, Jeanine. A family member of hers passed away and the funeral was at the church. Her grandmother was there and a few of her other relatives.

Gi, she looks so good!"

For no real reason, as nothing untoward had transpired between us, Jeanine and I hadn't been in touch for some time. I chalked up our distance to college years, really busy lives, and my intense focus in the church.

The minute that Mom said she spoke to Jeanine, I got this overwhelming sense that 'J' was *exactly* who I needed to speak with to get some advice about this therapy business.

There was a piece of me that needed to speak to someone who knew me "back in the day." Back in the days of Mr. Young Man and Frankie, and getting to know our older sister, and how all of that played into me running to the church and then running around *in* the church. Perhaps Jeanine could help me understand the emotional position I was in at that Moment.

Of course, I should talk to Jeanine.

"Ma, did she give you her new phone number?" In this period of time that we lost touch, I didn't even have a right number for J any longer."

"*Did she give me her number*?! Gi, she practically begged me to call you right then and there! I promised her that I would call you as soon as I got home and made sure that you two got reconnected. You really need to call her right away, Gigi. She was so excited to see me, and she had a million questions about where you were and how she could connect with you. She looked so, so good!"

That was the third time she told me how great Jeanine looked. That was precious and hilarious to me. Jeanine and my mother (as well as Jeanine's Mom, Cecilia, and I) had their own friendship over the years. It brought a smile to my heart thinking about how nice that "bumping into each other" Moment must have been for them both.

I called J within the half-hour.

It's hard to explain what that reconnection phone call was like. There was laughing, crying, and over talking (because we each had so much, we wanted to say to the other).

It was so incredibly great to reconnect. We must have been on the phone for at least the next three to four hours. As we effortlessly filled in the gaps of the last few years, it was as if no time had passed by.

NO time. None.

Not even a second.

There is something thoroughly healing about talking to someone who knows your *entire* back story. I didn't know it at the time, but to such a large extent I needed exactly that. I needed to speak with someone who knew me *then*.

And, who loved me then.

Jeanine needed that, too.

I explained in vivid detail to her all the events of the previous two years, including and up to Perla's death. I also confessed to her that I was starting to believe that it might be time for me to move back to the city.

I absolutely loved living in Central Jersey. I had 100% become a suburban girl. There was a piece of me that also knew that if I was really going to get better, I would have to face my past and the grief that I had run away from.

I told Jeanine that and asked her what she thought.

In true Jeanine fashion, she gave it to me straight – no chaser. *"Now Gi, I'm not going to lie, selfishly, I would love to have you back home, but you do what's right for you. I will say this. Listening to everything you just shared with me, your Pastor is right. You're not well, Gi. You're not doing well at all, and it sounds like you haven't been for some time.*

I absolutely think that what you need is to figure out how to heal. If that means coming home, then so be it, because Gi, you MUST heal. That part you must do."

I took the "coincidence" of my mother running into Jeanine as a message. I felt like God was trying to reach me and he knew he could do that through Jeanine. As I got back from Dr. Sleepy, I was 30 seconds from giving up. But God was in the mix, and I believe he was directing me. After talking with Jeanine, I decided that I was going to pack up my condo and go home.

It was time for me to face my demons, my past pain, and get serious about getting the help that I needed to heal.

It was time to get well.

SOON

Chapter 9

The Window

S<u>oon</u> brings what to your mind?

What do you think about when you hear the word *SOON*?

I'll tell you what *I* think.

I think, not yet but almost.

I think, not here but not far.

I think, hold on, it's just around the corner.

For me, the word "SOON" has promise to it.

It has a ring of possibility.

The sound of HOPE.

I had only been in my new condo (back in my old complex), for a short time. I still had several things in boxes that I hadn't unpacked.

But I was going home.

I was going back to the Bronx.

The plan was to put my things in storage (not the first time I had done that), and go home to heal.

When I say I was going home, I mean that I was *actually* going to move back into our childhood home.

The prospect of this felt all parts welcoming and a little scary at the same time. There's no place like home and that's the truth, but it would be the first time I lived in the house without Frankie.

Almost immediately after my father's passing, I moved back to New Jersey. After Dad's funeral, Mom sat us down and encouraged us to do what we thought we needed to do to get through those terrible days.

I knew what I needed to do. I needed to get out of the Bronx. By that time, New Jersey had certainly become a second home. I had done my college work there, my dearest sorority sisters were there, and I wanted to do my postgraduate work at Rutgers (and I wanted to do that work at Rutgers, New Brunswick) so going *back* to New Jersey for me right after Dad's passing made all the sense in the world.

Although I had been a member of the same church back in the Bronx, finding a congregation in Central Jersey was not hard at all. In fact, it was quite easy. I called the church office in early '93 and was given information about where the church met just outside of Somerset on Route 27.

At the first service, I came to love the brothers and sisters in Central Jersey with the fullness of my heart. I was so grateful to be in this very serene and quiet part of the Northeast that allowed me to get home back to the Bronx in less than 90 minutes.

I was grateful for Central Jersey, my friends, and church family that would always be in my heart. They still are to this day.

But it was time to go.

In the following weeks after my conversation with Jeanine, I started repacking my condo. Honestly, I was all over the place, but once I made the decision that I was moving back, I was ready to bounce.

However, during this time, one of my dearest friends and old roommates, Theresa, was getting married to another dear brother and friend, Aaron.

Theresa and I had been partners in the gospel during my time at Central and Aaron had always loved her. We have a basketful of hysterical memories about their dating life, and I wasn't going to miss their wedding for anything in the world.

The wedding was on a gorgeous day down in Princeton. It was beautiful and it felt good to have a bit of happiness after Perla's passing.

The night that I got home from Theresa and Aaron's wedding, I felt very flush. I hadn't been taking care of myself. By this time, I was deeply depressed and had been crying a lot. I chalked up this "feeling flushed" business to being overtired.

The next morning, I woke feeling quite ill, and the next day, I felt even worse than that. By the third day, I managed to get in my car and go to CVS for a thermometer. I had one somewhere, but it was packed in a box, and I didn't feel well enough to search for it.

I felt like I had a fever.

Sure enough, after taking my temperature, my fever was at 102F -- high for an adult. Oh boy. I know what this is. I wasn't coughing. I didn't have a cold, just this really high fever and incredible fatigue.

I went to bed that night and I woke up the next morning at about 5 AM. I don't remember this part very much because I was delirious and evidently in somewhat of a fever haze. Somehow, I managed to call my little sister, Gida.

I do remember her saying to me:

"Gi, you sound like you need some help."

People had been saying that to me a lot back then.

She asked if I had a thermometer. I remember saying that I did, and she admonished me to get it and take my temperature right then while she was on the phone.

I remember this, but I also remember thinking that this all happened in a dream.

But it was real. I was *really* sick.

When I read her that my temperature was at 104F, the sound of her voice changed.

Ordinarily, Gida is no alarmist, but this time she was alarmed.

"Gigi... *Gigi*... listen to me carefully. You must get to the emergency room. Now! Is there anybody that you could call? You CANNOT drive yourself. Are you hearing me?"

I heard her, but I was in a stupor.

I was feverish and confused but somehow, I managed to call a friend who lived close by. When my girlfriend arrived, I remember barely being able to stand and burning up with fever.

As she dropped me off at the front entrance of the emergency room, a nurse greeted me at the information desk and rushed me to an emergency nurse. The nurse took one look, grabbed my temperature, and took me straight to the back to be seen.

After collecting my insurance information, I was put in an emergency room bed and instantly hooked up to an IV.

I was having a Sarcoidosis attack, and this was the drill.

I had been diagnosed with Sarcoidosis a few years before (hence my concerns about this auto-immune disorder and hair loss).

Typically, what would happen in these attacks (I often called them episodes), was that either my lungs or kidneys would get inflamed.

This time, it was my kidneys, and I was sick as a dog.

I stayed in the emergency room patient area until late that night. The attending physician, who had treated me all day, came to say, "we're so sorry, Miss Gilliard, we are going to have to keep you."

Fan-freakin-tastic.

This would have been, over the course of the previous three years, my *fourth* hospital stay due to a Sarcoidosis related incident.

Here I was, in the middle of packing, getting my mind right about moving back to the Bronx, working on getting into therapy, and I land my fool self in the hospital again.

I was *not* enjoying myself.

The next morning, the phone began to ring in my hospital room as my relatives began calling. It was a series of relatives. First, Mom, then my sisters, and my cousins Tiffany and Butter called. Then, my Aunt Mena called, then Uncle Bob and my Cousin Joe-Joe, and Aunt To-To.

I had been on the phone with my family all morning. Between the nurses coming in and me running my mouth all morning, I was exhausted and began to drift off to sleep.

The phone rang once more, and it was Aunt Gracie.

My Aunt Gracie has a definitive way about her. Outside of my mother, who is our family matriarch, Aunt Gracie was like the second mama to everybody. All my Aunties have had a tremendous influence in my life. My Dad's eldest sister, Aunt Ynetha (Aunt "Letha"), is by far the most spiritually faithful individual I know. My Aunt Mena has a loving and protective spirit that is unmatched. Aunt Toto (her name is Patsy, but we call her Toni and Frankie called her Toto...so that stuck), taught me what being an "Auntie" should be about. She is one my dearest friends, a big sister, and sometimes also a second Mom.

But Aunt Gracie is the boss.

Even though she is the middle of my Dad's sisters, Aunt Gracie writes the law.

"Hi Auntie..."

"*Babbbbby...* What's the matter?"

Uh-oh.

Aunt Gracie is wise and has been through so many things herself. For whatever reason, she had it in her mind that morning that she was going to tell me what was all-the-way-good.

"Your Mom told me that you were thinking about coming home, is that true?"

I told her it was and that, ironically, I was in the middle of packing over the last couple of days and that I had gone to my girlfriend's wedding before I started feeling badly.

"Well, do you want to know what I think?"

My father's sisters are very funny. Aunt Gracie asked me if I wanted to know what she thought, but she knew full well that she didn't care if I wanted to know.

She was going to tell me either way!

"You have been going through a great deal, Gigi, for a great while now. It is past time for you to go home and get better. Your Mom has been so worried about you. We've been worried about you, and you need to heal."

If one more person told me I needed to heal…

Got it, God.

10-4. The message was clear.

So many messengers:

Perla, our ministry leader, Joey, Jeanine… and now Aunt Gracie.

It was time to go home.

I remained in the hospital for the next three days. The good doctors and nurses got my kidneys together.

I went back to my place to get ready to pack.

I was going to press my way back to the Bronx in the next two weeks. I worked things out with the management office, bought boxes, and arranged with my sister's very dear friend to come help me move.

The biggest piece of furniture I had was my long comfy couch that was definitely going into storage. A lot of my other furniture I was willing to part with. Outside of the couch and my clothes, I either gave or threw everything else away.

Within the next two weeks, I was coming across the George Washington Bridge back into New York City with all my earthly belongings stuffed into my little clown car.

There's a point on the George Washington Bridge when you cross over the border from New Jersey to New York.

On the other side of the crossing, I made a mental note that I was home.

Coming home was weird, but also felt really good.

While it was strange to sleep in my childhood bedroom, Mom and I had decided that I would take both bedrooms and the bathroom on the upper floor and turn it into my own small living quarters.

The plan was that I was going take over both rooms - - with one becoming my office or sitting room and the other one as my bedroom.

I had resigned from my job in Central Jersey so by the time I had moved back to the Bronx, I was not working.

I don't care how many therapists I needed to see, Gigi not working *was not going to work.* I've always been a workaholic and had done well (very well), in the learning and development space.

As such, it wasn't long before I got a new job at a major advertising firm in the city. I came on in an entry-level role and before long began running trainings for their on-boarding process. Shortly after, I was named the chair of their diversity and inclusion committee. It's funny to think about this now because the decision to take that chair role changed my life.

In that moment, though, I was just settling in to being back in the city.

Now remember:

The goal was to come home and heal. Perla said it, my Pastor said it, Aunt Gracie said it, and Jeanine said it.

As I told you, it was clear that God was talking to me. While I knew for certain that I did need to heal, being back home immediately made me think of boys.

Fight me.

Against my better judgment, I reached out to an old friend (all my therapists and coaches reading that last line are now screaming, in unison, "*NOOOOO!!!!!!*").

Oh, but yes. Hard eyeroll.

"Love addiction" would be the death of me.

It was the last thing I needed, but the comfort of yet another ill-timed relationship was what I reached for.

Someone that I knew (that had been interested in me while I was dating Mr. Young Man all those years ago), found out that I was back in New York City. We went out on a couple of dinner and movie dates and found that we were both still single and both in similar stations in life.

Before long, without even realizing it, we had become a couple. We would go on to date for the next 12 years and I would add one more behemoth of a mammoth size hurt to have to heal from.

In the meantime, though, with renewed insurance benefits, I resumed my quest for a therapist.

Jeanine and I were back to hanging out on a regular basis, talking two or three times a day, and I had begun attending a new church.

I was well aware that I had unfinished business to attend to with my emotions.

I repeated the process that I learned back in Jersey. I called my new company's EAP line and got connected with someone who acted like a concierge, much like

Joey (but nothing like Joey... I loved Joey), but the new EAP guide came *all the way* through.

****

I was given the name of a male therapist on the upper east side of Manhattan.

The EAP representative forwarded his profile and I loved what I read.

He was a person of color, a native New Yorker, and he specialized in grief, loss, and trauma.

This was intriguing.

We set up a meeting. While I was nervous (very nervous, in fact, after my delicate girl at Rutgers and Dr. Sleepy), I actually felt optimistic.

When I arrived for our first appointment and sat down across from him, I liked him immediately.

He had salsa music playing in his office and during that first visit all we did was talk about music and growing up in New York in the 70s and 80s.

Looking back on it now, I see what he was doing.

He was connecting with me. He was allowing me to *feel him out.* It was brilliant and I'll always be grateful for that.

We spent the next few weeks listening to music and talking as old friends.

He asked what I wanted to get out of our time together. I shared what I wanted.

Early on, most of our conversations were just laughing about the past (we were nearly the same age) and getting to know each other.

One session, he asked me to tell him about some of my earliest memories of loving someone.

It was an interesting exercise, but it had a point.

He followed up with some other significant questions and showed great interest in my family history. My relationship with Frankie, my Mom, my siblings, and God were really on his mind.

He sent me home with an exercise the following week. The exercise was very specific and required me to bring up some very detailed memories about the first time I remembered feeling hurt or sadness in a relationship.

When we got back together and I shared with him my responses, he replied:

"Do you see, Mija?"

Oh my. He called me "Mija" like Perla.

I was so moved.

"Do you see how that very first incident is connected to how you felt about leaving people and people leaving you? Do you see how the way that very early incident played out developed some expectations from you about your Dad? And how those expectations are connected on some level to how you felt about Mr. Young Man? And ultimately, how you have moved in so many of your relationships?

I did see it.

I saw it so very clearly.

The point he was making was stunningly clear and I had never seen it before. I had never made the connection. It was so blatant that I was astonished how I had never made the correlation until just that moment. I think I said something like,

"Oh, my gracious... I never thought about that before. I would have never put that together. It makes so much complete sense. Wow. Wow. Wow."

Clarity.

What I needed, to at least begin the healing, was clarity. Clarity was the gift I didn't know I needed.

The clarity I felt in that moment almost frightened me. It was almost as if we were sitting at a large table working on a 2,000-piece jigsaw puzzle, and in this one conversation the edges of the puzzle all started to fit.

I knew in that Moment that I would need to take time to figure out the other puzzle pieces so that I could see the entire picture.

Suddenly, I now had the frame.

Wow.

It was as if for many years I had been locked in a dark room with no air and there were a set of heavy curtains against one wall. All the time that I had spent in this dark room just staring at curtains, wishing for air, there sat a wall of wide picture windows just on the other side of the curtains.

In all my life, it had never occurred to me to pull back the curtains and expose the window. Without the guidance I didn't have the language or the mindset to know how.

All this time, I have been locked in this room with no air because I needed someone to help me discover the window. Someone to help me gain the clarity.

This window into my past, into my original trauma, and into my thinking patterns allowed me to see the cycles of my decisions.

The more we talked, the wider the window opened in my mind. The curtains were fully drawn and tied back, the sun began to stream in, and I would never be able to unsee the truth about myself again.

The clarity that I received that morning provided a feeling of relief that I can describe as synonymous only with hope.

Hope.

For the first time in years, I felt hopeful.

I felt like I had been given a key to a great mystery in my own life. This key would help me unlock and decipher many more points of clarity about myself, my view of God, the way I saw the world, the way I saw men, the way I experience people, and so much more.

I'm not going to be overly dramatic and tell you that I was cured or healed in that moment. That would be a lie. _I was not._

I wasn't healed, and, in fact, I am _still_ healing. However, I realized that this kind of talking things through, this kind of piecing things together, (with the help of licensed mental health professional), is what it means to do the work. There would be years of more work to be done. I am still working on myself in therapy today – _even as I pen this._

This window of clarity became an amulet of great understanding. On some level, in that moment of crystallization, I got it.

I realized that there was so much more to uncover, but I got it.

I got who I was, and I got *why* I was.

I was beautiful.

God had made me so. God has made *you*, so.

And on my way to getting well.

What Auntie Wants You to Know

Chapter 10

What Auntie Wants You To Know

A s I was finishing up this book my therapist said, *"Of course finishing this book is hard. You're sharing and opening up about layers of grief of loss in the middle of… grief and loss."*

#Facts.

Her comment made me think about the first thing I wanted to leave you with.

The pandemic hit my family hard. Very hard.

However, I will not arrogantly assert that our family had it any harder than anyone else. We did not. We know that so many other families, upon families, suffered loss upon loss.

What I will say is that in the stretch of time that I decided to share all of this with you all…so much more transpired. So much more took place, and I suffered so much more grief and loss. But even in that I know that I am not the only one (by far) to have done so.

Grief is not a respecter of persons and the pain from loss is not a bigot, but rather happily doles out equal opportunity heartache. I've just had a lot of it.

A lot of heartache.

A great deal of loss.

An inordinate number of goodbyes.

I know that the pain I've felt from these losses, from hard goodbyes, has been, in part, compounded by the way that I attach.

And I DO attach. I am aware.

For all of the days that I struggled with emotional wellness and mental illness the only place that I could find solace or a balm, a real salve, was through understanding that God was a friend that would never leave me.

I came to understand that with God there was a healing power. Ultimately, it was this power that led me to find the resources that could help me decipher how to process the pain and hurt from trauma that had gone unresolved.

Now the thing about life and sadness, and grief and loss, and work and bills, and pressure and society, and the news and racism, and pandemics and politics, and colonialism and hunger and global warming and wars, is that life's maladies, both big and small, can overwhelm us to the point of sickness.

But for me, having decided that I believed in Jesus Christ and his message was the very thing that gave me the strength to fight to get to the other side of the bridge of "get well soon."

It was (and is) my relationship with God that helps me process and heal from hurt, and grief, and sadness, and depression, and loss to get to the other side.

For me, understanding that God wanted me to feel better, that **HE** wanted me to heal and get well soon was the very thing that drove me to get help.

It is not my intention to push my faith down your throat. It is simply my desire to do just that – share my faith – and how that faith has guided me; protected me. That's the first thing I wanted you know.

That was the first thing. Now, for the second.

Have you ever seen the movie, *Close Encounters of The Third Kind?*

I have five all-time favorite movies. Of these five, *Close Encounters of The Third Kind,* released in 1977, is by far my all-time favorite movie.

My dad, when he was alive, was a sci-fi buff. He was the quintessential Trekkie, and even owned a telescope to watch the stars and all things universe (I totally believe he was looking for unidentified flying objects). This perhaps may be where I get it from because I too, have an appetite for sci-fi. I believe that the God of the universe, the God of *this* world, could FOR CERTAIN, be the God of many other worlds as well. Not sure.

But *Close Encounters of The Third Kind* is my favorite movie because if you've seen it, you might remember that Richard Dreyfuss' character (Roy Neary) had become obsessed with this sensation of being compelled towards something much bigger than he.

In his character's case, one night after a brief but very powerful encounter with a strange UFO (unidentified flying object), 'Roy', from that moment on became fixated with getting to a certain location. He somewhat had an image of this location in mind, but had no idea where that location was, or what any of it was intended to mean. The image of the location was a large wide mountain with deep grooves along its side. In his mind, the prompting, (though powerful and intense), was very ambiguous. He wasn't entirely sure *why* he kept thinking about this particular place and initially he didn't even know that what he was seeing in his mind's eye was even a place.

He kept thinking about this image of a "thing", but he had no idea what this thing was. Before long he, and other characters in the movie that had experienced the same encounter with this UFO on that same night were driven to this strange ambiguous place. Much of the plot of the movie chronicles how this group of people who shared this experience with one another all somehow, in a telepathic, "way-that-couldn't-be-explained," needed to find themselves at this mountain.

These people were being pushed and compelled and often couldn't sleep at night because they were so compelled by this image. They knew, that for some reason, they _had_ to get there.

I was 10 in 1977. But even that young I remember feeling a kindred sentiment with those characters. I felt a prompting, a pushing. A drive _to do a thing_. One of my favorite young (but oh so very wise) pastors, Jerry Flowers, describes it as an "unction." It wasn't until about 2006 that I realized that this lifelong prodding was less about something I need to do as it was more about something I need to _say_.

I've always written. I've considered myself a writer since a child. I've long since believed that what I needed to say, whatever message I had to deliver, was to be delivered on paper. I believe that the beginnings of that 'something to say' were found in the pages of the *Loud Brown Round Girl*. Thank you so much to those of you who took the time to read that fledgling work. However, just a short while after I came up with the *Loud Brown Round Girl* title, the title for this book was dropped in my spirit.

As I mentioned to you earlier, it happened that one morning when I was standing in my kitchen, broken hearted, I looked up at my counter and I saw 2 coffee mugs sitting together.

Cup number one read, "Hello Beautiful," and cup number two read, "Get Well Soon."

From that very moment until this, I knew for certain that the unction I felt my whole life was the intention for me to use and say, "*all my words.*"

That phrase, "*say all your words*" is something that those in my inner circle have heard me utter many times. Say all your words.

But because of my faith, I also believed that if you were going to speak any words, they needed to be worthy. In fact, there the Scripture message in Jeremiah 15:19 says exactly that. "… if you utter worthy, not worthless, words, you will be my spokesman."

It was critical for me to "say all my words," but more important for those words to be worthy. This was the charge; this was the calling. When the calling became clear,

I began to pray and ask God for the specifics. What was it *exactly* that he wanted me to say? The morning of the cups (and two other mornings like it in the future) it became crystal clear to me what I was supposed to say.

Thinking back about the story of the "dash," I want desperately to ensure that my life on earth is unarguably focused on serving and helping others. I knew for sure that it was incumbent upon me to take that which was the darkest, most embarrassing, most difficult, and most painful and share it with the world in a way that could prayerfully help just one individual feel seen, heard, and understood.

It was also my desire to give even just one individual the tiniest sliver of hope if that hope could help them to get well; if that hope could help them see, even, that they *needed* to get well; if that hope could help them to feel better …or maybe even save the life.

I realize what a lofty goal and prayer that is. However, like Richard Dreyfuss' character in that movie, I couldn't help myself - - even if I tried. It was as if God wouldn't let me rest.

With everything in me I believe that God allowed some of the things to happen in my life so that in 2021, specifically right now in this moment in time, I would be equipped to share these things with you.

I believe that God waited until *now* where I would be more emotionally equipped, more developed in the maturation of my personality and my character; more established in business and resources in order to share with you this message.

Openly and unashamedly, I do pray that some of you, even one of you, can read some of these words and find yourself through your own dark tunnel of pain. I pray that some of you, even *one* of you, might consider getting help through the discipline of therapeutic counseling and care from a mental health professional (if you need it). I also pray that in some way my faith in God and the hope that I found in Him might encourage you, even if it is just one of you as well.

Finally, I am fully aware that so many of you have been through far, far, far worse than I have. My heart is full of compassion for you. I may not know your story but I'm praying for you… and I'm praying that you can be okay… I'm praying that somehow you know today that you are not alone.

I also pray that you got a chuckle or two out of all of this, because it is my consistent desire to continue to show up as your ridiculous auntie.

Thank you for being on this journey with me. Thank you for the honor of your company and the gift of your time. Thank you so very much.

It's been my pleasure to be with you again in these pages.

There are some resources on the final pages here that you may find helpful. The times that we are living in are like no other. The weight of a pandemic, friends, and family that we have lost, the struggle of being in our homes for almost 2 years, the pressure to not "get canceled" at every turn, the economy, politics, racism, violence, war - - *relationships*.

It has been a lot.

If you need help, if you need someone to talk to – *please* reach out to someone.

Please get help, please work on getting well if need be.

Please take care of yourself.

Oh, …and one last thing.

Next time, I wanna tell you a story about lizards, leviathans, scoundrels, and weasels - - you might want to come back for that - - you might find it interesting… and *entertaining*.

wink

Until we meet again…
let's be well, and let's be well to each other.

((Hugs))

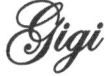

<u>Citations</u>

Holy Bible. New International Version, 2021, https://www.bible.com/.com/niv/

Resources

Help is available

Speak with someone today
National Suicide Prevention Lifeline
Hours: Available 24 hours. Languages: English, Spanish.

800-273-8255

Emergency: 911
National Domestic Violence Hotline:
1- 800-799-7233
National Suicide Prevention Lifeline:
1-800-273-TALK (8255)
National Hopeline Network:
1-800-SUICIDE (800-784-2433)
Crisis Text Line: Text "DESERVE" TO 741-741
**Lifeline Crisis Chat (Online live
messaging):** https://suicidepreventionlifeline.org/chat/
Self-Harm Hotline: 1-800-DONT CUT (1-800-366-8288)
Planned Parenthood Hotline: 1-800-230-PLAN (7526)
American Association of Poison Control Centers: 1-800-222-1222
**National Council on Alcoholism & Drug Dependency Hope
Line:** 1-800-622-2255
National Crisis Line - Anorexia and Bulimia: 1-800-233-4357
GLBT Hotline: 1-888-843-4564
TREVOR Crisis Hotline: 1-866-488-7386
AIDS Crisis Line: 1-800-221-7044
Veterans Crisis Line: https://www.veteranscrisisline.net
TransLifeline: https://www.translifeline.org - 877-565-8860
Suicide Prevention Wiki: http://suicideprevention.wikia.com

PLEASE NOTE:

These resources are intended as exploration aids and search recommendations for research only. Please fully and appropriately vet health care providers that best suit your needs. Seek counsel from ONLY certified and licensed mental health professionals with proven credentials.

Helpful Resources for the Black & Brown Community:

Reginald Howard
https://reginaldahoward.com/podcast/

AFFIRM
https://www.justdavia.com/podcast

The Bodyful Black Girl Podcast
https://jennifersterling.com/podcast

Melanin and Mental Health/ Between Sessions
https://www.melaninandmentalhealth.com/category/between-sessions/
http://blackyouthproject.com/6-mental-health-awareness-podcasts-and-shows-for-black-women/

https://therapyforblackgirls.com/

Resources for All - Helpful Online Resources:

Dr. Ramani Durvasula
http://doctor-ramani.com/
https://www.youtube.com/channel/UC9Qixc77KhCo88E5muxUjmA

Tamie Joyce, Life Coach
https://www.tamiemcoaching.com/
https://www.youtube.com/channel/UCfVEc3ET8BnI5ecvKF5-cEQ

https://www.betterhelp.com/
https://www.talkspace.com/

Made in the USA
Middletown, DE
22 November 2021

53164089R00179